In their own words:

THREE MARITIMERS EXPERIENCE THE GREAT WAR, 1914–1918

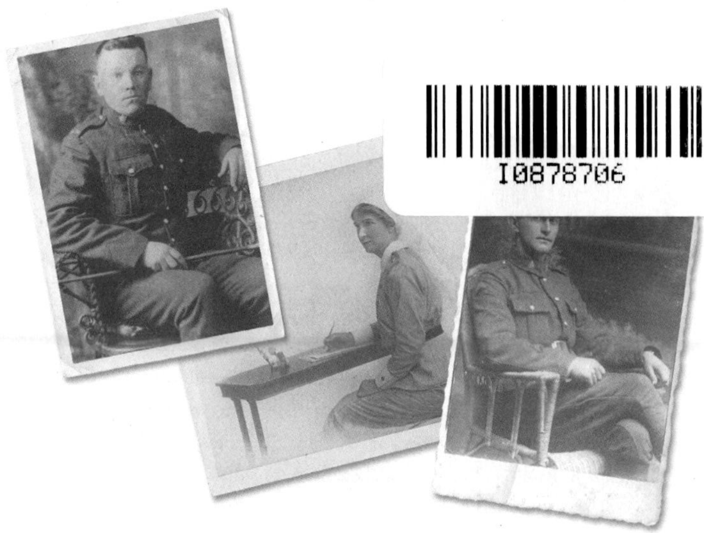

Edited by Ross N. Hebb

NIMBUS PUBLISHING
NIMBUS.CA

Nimbus Publishing Limited
3660 Strawberry Hill Street, Halifax, NS, B3K 5A9
(902) 455-4286 nimbus.ca

Printed and bound in Canada
NB1321

MIX
Paper from responsible sources
FSC www.fsc.org FSC® C013916

Cover and interior design: Andrew Herygers

Library and Archives Canada Cataloguing in Publication

In their own words (Halifax, N.S.)
In their own words / edited by Ross Hebb.
Includes index.
Issued in print and electronic formats.
ISBN 978-1-77108-670-7 (softcover).—ISBN 978-1-77108-671-4 (HTML)

1. Poole, Eugene A.—Correspondence. 2. Balloch, Pauline—Correspondence. 3. Heckbert, Herry—Correspondence. 4. Soldiers—Maritime Provinces—Correspondence. 5. Nurses—Maritime Provinces—Correspondence. 6. World War, 1914-1918—Personal narratives,Canadian. 7. World War, 1914-1918—Maritime Provinces. 8. Personal correspondence. I. Hebb, Ross N., editor II. Poole, Eugene A. .Correspondence. Selections. III. Balloch, Pauline . Correspondence. Selections. IV. Heckbert, Herry . Correspondence. Selections. V. Title.

D640.A2I5 2018 940.4'8171 C2018-902908-0
C2018-902909-9

Canada NOVA SCOTIA Canada Council for the Arts Conseil des arts du Canada

Nimbus Publishing acknowledges the financial support for its publishing activities from the Government of Canada, the Canada Council for the Arts, and from the Province of Nova Scotia. We are pleased to work in partnership with the Province of Nova Scotia to develop and promote our creative industries for the benefit of all Nova Scotians.

Dedicated to the memory of my father, Ralph Whitfield Hebb
(F79081, Royal Canadian Engineers),

and great-great-uncle, John Garfield Hebb
(477395, The Royal Canadian Regiment),

Canadians who, in their own generation, walked the fields of France and Flanders armed with Bren gun and Ross rifle so that I, in my generation, could return armed with only a camera and a deep sense of awe and appreciation

CONTENTS

INTRODUCTION

We no longer write letters like the ones found in this volume. Letter writing is a dying art. With the passing of cursive handwriting, the very alphabet in which these letters were scripted is also disappearing. We live in the age of instant, abbreviated communication. We send texts, tweets, posts, messages, and, if we have the time, email. Although much has been gained with this progress, much has also been lost. The letters in this book come to us from a different time, offering us a glimpse into a different era of communication. They are one hundred years old, yet their originality and vitality are striking. Though far from home, the men and women who penned these letters carried on sustained conversations with loved ones for years. The conversations were organic, lively, and evolving. The letters do not simply communicate facts; they also paint descriptive pictures of places, events, and people. They express anxiety, fear, hope, and love without emojis and downloaded pics. The writers communicated using words, and they chose their words carefully. The letters also clearly convey the unique personality of each of their authors. The distinct teasing of a younger sister by an older brother, the concern of a daughter for an elderly parent, and the lovesick cry of a groom separated from his new bride—all this and much more come to us through these letters and across time. Perhaps a challenge is in order: once you have finished this volume, review a year's worth of your Facebook posts, compare them to a year of these letters, and ask yourself who has best succeeded in communicating a year in their life?

These letters do more than express the spirit of their authors, for they also transport us through time. They take us back to the way we were here in Maritime Canada one hundred years ago. We learn of life in Bridgetown, Nova Scotia; Centreville, New Brunswick; and Summerside, Prince Edward Island—typical of Maritime communities of the time. The Maritimes was not then an area of devastated rural communities stymied by unemployment and bereft of young families. The majority of the people had not left the family farms and small villages for the region's few cities or for jobs elsewhere in the Dominion. Most of the population was rural, the most vital transportation links were by train, and the mail travelled relatively quickly and efficiently. As we learn from the letters, young women were needed as school teachers in Nova Scotia, and men were required as farmhands in New Brunswick and as fishermen in Prince Edward Island. Moreover, Maritimers fed themselves: they farmed, they fished, and they hunted. As the letters reveal, there were apples and moose in the Annapolis Valley, potatoes and maple syrup in the St. John River valley, and fish and lobsters in the waters off Summerside. It is true that plumbing was still outdoors and electricity had not yet arrived in most areas, but the telephone had already begun to ring in Maritime homes. The overwhelming impression left by these letters, however, is that life in Maritime Canada was good. Although they lacked the conveniences and the comforts of today, families were happy. As these letters show, relationships between young men and women and with their parents and siblings were strong, close, and vital. We cannot help but conclude that the ties that bound families and communities together were at least as strong and enduring then as they are today.

This book presents three unique and distinct sets of letters. What sets the volume apart, however, is that it contains not just a few letters from individuals who lived through the First World War, but all the letters they wrote about their wartime experience. The Eugene Poole collection ranks as genuinely rare among Canadian Great War correspondence: the letters of a young man who joined up in August 1914, served the entire war, and lived to return! Of the thirty-three thousand men in the First Contingent of the Canadian Expeditionary Force (CEF), more than five thousand were killed at the Second Battle of Ypres in April 1915. Eugene survived. And he was no rear-echelon man serving far behind the lines: as his letters attest, he served at the front, and penned many letters in dugouts under shellfire. His gunshot wound reminds us of the grave dangers he faced. Eugene Poole also survived Passchendaele. Moreover, unlike some First Contingent men, he did not enjoy several months' furlough back in Canada—indeed, he received no great amount of leave over the course of the entire war. Whether we regard him as a statistical anomaly or as protected by a higher power, Poole survived the entire war, writing to his parents and sisters throughout. We are now privileged to have his letters to read. They are a treasure.

Nursing Sister Pauline Ballock's correspondence is a very different find. Although several thousand Canadian women, many of them Maritimers, served as nursing sisters during the Great War, they have not yet received the attention or the credit they deserve. Only a few diaries and even fewer letters survive, among them those of Ina Lockhart of Petitcodiac, New Brunswick, and the full (published) diary of Clare Gass of Shubenacadie, Nova Scotia. Amazingly and fortunately, however, we have a whole year's worth of correspondence from Pauline Balloch to her parents that cover her entire war experience. These nurses—called sisters, although they were not in any religious order—were a unique group. Once they had joined the Canadian Army Medical Corps (CAMC), the Canadian army uniquely granted them officer status (as lieutenants) and a distinct powder-blue uniform. These nursing sisters not only outranked most of the men they cared for; they were also older, usually in their thirties, and single, when the war broke out. As such, they represented a small but important emerging cohort in pre-war Canada. Trained in the hospitals of large Canadian cities such as Montreal or in the "Boston states" (including New York), they were something new in society: educated, unattached, and financially independent women!

What has been said of Claire Gass applies equally to Pauline Balloch (and Ina Lockhart): she "went to war as a patriotic Canadian, a dutiful daughter, a devout Anglican, a loving sister, a dear friend, an adventurer, a romantic—and a nurse."[1] What can be added is that Balloch, like the men who served, did not return unchanged by the experience. Her letters provide hints of her evolving transformation. Interestingly, unlike both Ina Lockhart and Clare Gass, who remained single, Pauline did marry upon her return to Canada. In June 1921, at age forty, Pauline wed widower Willard L. Carr, a man almost twenty years her senior. One is tempted to speculate that the marriage was a perfectly simple arrangement between two rational individuals whereby Pauline would nurse her aging husband until death did them part—indeed, Willard died two years later, in 1923. Such an arrangement was proper, dignified, and caring, all traits that the nursing sisters embodied and practised throughout their lives. Pauline would never remarry.

Harry Heckbert's letters are unique, too, but for an unusual and unexpected reason. Harry did not want to go to war, and by late 1917 he had still not joined up. Despite years of political speeches, weekly sermons, and unremitting societal pressure, including intense recruitment drives in 1916, Harry had not volunteered. Harry was no coward, nor was he alone. Like tens of thousands of other Canadians, including thousands of Maritimers, who chose to work on the farms and fishing boats and in the mines and factories feeding and supplying the national war effort, Harry was not convinced he should go to war. Moreover, of all those who served in the CEF, fully 51 percent had been born in the United Kingdom, but Harry was a native born Maritimer and, like the rest of his family, a fisherman. Fishing is labour intensive and requires men, and Harry had remained home and fished with his brothers and father. By 1917, however, manpower was desperately needed. The empire of which Canada was a part was in a struggle to the death, and men had to be found. Loss-

1 Susan Mann, ed., *The War Diary of Clare Gass: 1915–1918* (Montreal; Kingston, ON: McGill-Queen's University Press, 2000), xiii.

es at the front were not being made good through volunteers, and Canada's ability to continue the fight was at stake. Military conscription was debated, contested, voted on in December 1917, and then enforced in early 1918. Harry's, then, is the voice of the conscripted, of those who, however reluctantly, went to war nonetheless. His is a perspective often overlooked and forgotten, but Harry's story also needs to be recorded and preserved—in his own words.

A COMMENT ON SOURCES

The sights, sounds, and smells of Fredericton's Boyce Farmers Market are replicated in numerous farmers' markets throughout the Maritimes. These markets are a tribute to earlier, simpler days, and an affirmation of the quality and value of locally grown Maritime products. On a crisp autumn morning in 2014, amidst the mingled smells of Vietnamese cooking and barbequed German sausages, I happened to encounter Peggy Godsoe. She mentioned that she possessed some letters written by her grandfather, Eugene Poole, who had served in the Great War. As a result of Peggy's generosity, this singular collection of fifty letters by a man who joined in August 1914 and lived to return in 1919 can now see the light of day. The provenance of the letters is clear: the entire collection was preserved by Eugene's mother; in turn, Eugene's youngest sister Leila, who was only fourteen at the time he left for war, shared them with her niece Peggy in the early 1980s.

Interest in their roots is an ongoing passion for many, and it is often the case that folks take up their own genealogical research upon retirement. Such was the situation for Bob Balloch of Riverview, New Brunswick. In the course of his investigations, Bob discovered the letters of his great aunt, Nursing Sister Pauline Balloch. Learning of my interest in such matters, on his own initiative Bob called me, and the very next day hand-delivered coloured photocopies of all of the thirty-three letters Pauline wrote from April 1917 to April 1918—the entire period of her war service from the time she joined until she returned to Canada to care for her ailing mother. Pauline wrote almost exclusively to her parents in Centreville, New Brunswick. Her letters reveal a wartime experience that differed markedly from that of Eugene Poole, and are singularly interesting. To see the war from a more mature person's perspective and from a woman's vantage point is both refreshing and revealing, and Pauline offers insights without which we would all be the poorer.

Maritimers are known not only for their generosity, but for their hospitality as well. Kay Wall of New Annan, just outside Summerside, Prince Edward Island, is a case in point. Hearing of my interest in Great War letters, Kay emailed me in June of 2012. When I travelled to the Island in early September, she not only was willing to lend me the entire binder of her grandfather Harry Heckbert's letters, but welcomed me into her home and fed me supper as well! Kay's photocopies come compliments of her first cousin. In September 1917, Harry married Iva Mae Currie. Upon being conscripted for service the following spring, Harry wrote his new bride frequently, sometimes daily, penning sixty-four letters between April 1918 and February 1919. Harry spoke for thousands of other conscripted Maritime men—seven thousand from New Brunswick alone—whose voices are seldom heard in the story of the Great War. Despite the acknowledged justice of the war, for these men and their extended families, their "immediate concerns were of maintaining ancestral lands and fishing grounds or struggling in disparate ways to advance their collective rights."[2] Harry's letters exude loneliness, homesickness, and a newly married groom's lovesick heart at being separated from his pregnant wife. His letters also reveal a personal metamorphosis from reluctant conscript to determined soldier. By October 1918, Harry was ready and determined to go to France and do his bit. The Armistice came into effect shortly before he arrived, and Harry was spared the agonies and horrors of combat. Fortunately, and unlike many others, Harry got to return home to his wife and the child he had not yet met.

2 Andrew Theobald, *The Bitter Harvest of War: New Brunswick and the Conscription Crisis of 1917* (Fredericton, NB: Goose Lane Editions, 2008), 98.

ACKNOWLEDGEMENTS

Readers interested in learning more about the three individuals whose correspondence appears in this volume are urged to consult the website of Library and Archives Canada (LAC). Once there, under the heading of "Military Heritage," search "Soldiers of the First World War" to obtain each person's sign-up or "attestation papers." Since my earlier work, *Letters Home: Maritimers and the Great War*, LAC thankfully has received sufficient funding to embark on the process of digitizing the entire file of each Canadian soldier and nurse of the Great War. Initially projected to take a couple of years, it now appears the process will run almost the same length as the war itself: four full years more or less. The internet accessibility of the entire Great War file of each person, ranging in length from several to, in some cases, almost one hundred pages of information, represents an extraordinary advancement in the availability of our nation's heritage. Great War historians, families, and genealogists should be duly appreciative.

Access to such information demands understanding on the part of those who read the files. There is also the need for discretion in their usage and dissemination. The files normally include each individual's complete military and medical record. As well as learning where and when and in which unit one's grandfather served while overseas, the files also tell us if he was ever insubordinate to authority and punished for such behaviour. This was not unusual for men who signed up, as they said, "to fight, not soldier." Men who were used to making their own decisions and finding their own way often found it difficult to take orders—especially if, as was the case in later years, the order giver was younger and inexperienced. In reading such files, the general rule seems to be: the longer a man served, the more likely instances of friction with authority arose. Don't be surprised if your grandfather was one such man.

The medical records hold their own stories and their own secrets. As well as seeing exactly what your great-uncle's teeth looked like on his dental chart, you will also learn of everything for which he was hospitalized. Fevers, nasty skin infections, the 'flu, which was often lethal in 1918–19, and a variety of socially transmitted diseases are all recorded. The general statistical estimate is that at least 30 percent of the CEF contracted and were treated for some sort of STD during their war service. It is best to treat such personal discoveries with empathy and understanding. Single, young, lonely, and far from home, the men understandably sought connections that were often intimate. Once exposed to the front and the random death and dismemberment it entailed, the thought of returning repeatedly to the forward area not surprisingly lowered the men's caution and discretion. If you thought it unlikely that you would be returning home whole enough to be marriageable or even at all, then the urge to experience sexual intimacy before you were dismembered or literally blown to bits became a calculated risk many undertook. The flip side also has to be understood in the proper context: married men and the very principled who wrote of their efforts not to be unfaithful should not be viewed as holier-than-thou prudes, but as men struggling to maintain their principles in an environment unimaginable both to us and to those on the home front at the time.

In addition to acknowledging the advances at LAC, I wish to mention two other workers in the field of Great War research. Curtis Mainville has spent untold hours researching New Brunswick's newspapers from the Great War period. His assistance in ferreting out letters home from New Brunswick's Great War nurses of the CAMC and other services is expanding the understanding of this under-researched aspect of our history. In the former Dominion, now province, of Newfoundland and Labrador, I am grateful to archivist Craig Tucker of the province's museum, The Rooms, who has readily shared the unique experience of Newfoundlanders in the Great War. The Great War exhibit in The Rooms is of a very high calibre, and includes the story of the island's many nurses. The permanent exhibit uniquely manages to communicate the reality of the war as consuming the attention and effort of everyone on the home front as well as of the men overseas.

In conclusion, I would be remiss if I did not again acknowledge the assistance of the Canon W.A. Morris scholarship of Halifax. This funding has enabled me to continue my Great War research with particular emphasis on nurses. Their ongoing support and encouragement are most appreciated. Finally, I would like to thank freelance copy editor Barry Norris for his assistance; his efforts resulted in a tighter and more readable text.

THE CHARACTERS

Eugene Atwood POOLE
Born: July 10, 1891
Birthplace: Paradise, Nova Scotia
Parents: father: Frank J. Poole; mother: Foretta (Bockman) Poole
Siblings: Vera, Ida, Leila
Joined: September 27, 1914; discharged August 1919 (serving an amazing 3 years, 1 month in France)
Unit: Canadian Corps, Cyclist Division

Pauline Douglas BALLOCH
Born: February 23, 1882
Birthplace: Centreville, New Brunswick
Parents: father: Robert Wilmot Balloch; mother: Alice L. (Garden) Balloch
Siblings: Guy, Jack
Joined: May 2, 1917
Unit: Canadian Army Medical Corps

Harry HECKBERT
Born: May 3, 1887
Birthplace: Summerside, Prince Edward Island
Parents: father: Rufus A. Heckbert; mother: Eliza J. (Johnson) Heckbert
Siblings: Ella, Fred, Lena, Bruce, Florence, William, Earl
Married: Iva Mae Currie, September 5, 1917
Conscripted: March 23, 1918
Unit: First Depot Battalion, Nova Scotia Reserve; (in France) The Royal Canadian Regiment

Eugene A. Poole

OF BRIDGETOWN, NOVA SCOTIA

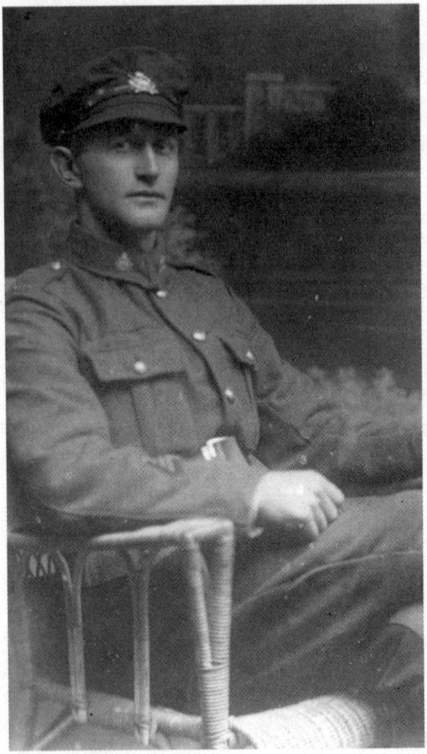

Eugene Poole seated early in the war.

Eugene Poole was very anxious to get to the war. In August 1914, he was twenty-four years old and had grown up in Bridgetown, Nova Scotia. He listed his profession as "machinist" on his attestation papers" or sign-up sheet. His parents' eldest child and only son, Eugene had three sisters: Vera, Ida, and Lelia. Eugene was also a member of the 69th Regiment of Militia.

It is this last piece of information that explains his presence at Valcartier military camp in Quebec in late August. Each province/military district had been asked to send a small contingent of trained militia men to the newly created camp at Valcartier. War had been declared only three weeks earlier, and Eugene was already in and on his way. Britain had asked for a contingent of twenty-five thousand men, and Canada was enthusiastic in its reply. Hoping to be accepted as a member of the First Contingent, Eugene writes his sister, speaking of his duties, his worries about passing the medical exams, and of the excitement, chaos, and disappointments experienced by the mass of "men" clamouring to get overseas.

August 29, 1914
Valcartier Camp, Quebec

Dear Sister,

I have not much to write but will fill in a few lines while I have the time. It is raining out tonight and bids fair to become a dismal day; on the morrow my duties as Orderly Sergt begin at 12 o'clock tomorrow. I do not relish it very much as it ties one to the camp and keeps a person always listening for the calls. There is a lot of sick feeling fellows alright—a lot of them not passing the physical exam. I have a cold which is not very nice, but I think I will get by the finals all right; would certainly hate to get thrown down now. We have not our Sergt's mess yet, but will have it now the first of the week; we have pretty good fare though for army life.

A woman was found the other day masquerading as a man, she was sent to prison. Another man felt so bad that they did not pass him he foolishly cut his throat. There was some talk of us going by way of Saint John, so your going to the landing was not too foolish. Fred and I tried to get leave Wednesday night of our departure but as we had a session before us they would not let us off. But we should not worry, it's all over now. Wait till the sun shines Nellie and Johnnie comes marching home.

Yours lovingly,
Sergt E. A. Poole No 8 Company 3rd Provincial Battalion

Writing a month later, Eugene tells his father of the marvel the Valcartier military camp has become. He also comments on problems at the camp, of mock battles, a possible transfer, and the larger-than-life Canadian minister of militia, Colonel Sam Hughes.

September 18,
Valcartier, Quebec

Dear Father,

The notice of no more mail to be sent out has been cancelled but the "tent city" presents a view which I would never have believed possible for any camp to attain. I have been very disappointed in the organization of the N.S. volunteers, due however to the small enlistment and the stubbornness of Col Andrews. Col. S. Hughes paraded us one day and gave us a straight sensible talk, which anyone could tell was sincere; he showed some of the officers up like mere school-boys. I have been offered two stripes in the Victoria Rifles of Canada [based in Montreal] and I am going to get with them; they are a fine lot of fellows to a man. E. Jeffries and G. Mason have joined them. We had a wonderful sham battle yesterday. I was scout for a party of the Vics (segt commanding scouts). I ran into a body of the enemy and laid for half an hour under a thick copse—could have touched several of them at times! I just came off 24 hr guard duty tonight. Some ceremony. I am still in the 69th detachment,

Yours lovingly, Sergt E. A. Poole

In early October 1914, the First Contingent of thirty-three thousand troops sailed for England. At the time, it was the largest single troop crossing of the Atlantic in history. Despite all the disappointed volunteers turned down at their medicals, Canada ended up sending thousands more than Britain had originally requested. The crossing took eleven days, and the troops disembarked at Plymouth instead of Southampton as planned. The logistics of war were not working smoothly at this early date. Eugene tells his dad of the warm welcome the Canadians received and of how he longed to do his part in a "just cause."

October 20,
Plymouth, England

Dear Father,

After a beautiful trip over we swung into Plymouth a week ago tomorrow and have been at anchor in the harbour ever since. It has just been officially announced that we disembark tomorrow morning. The intentions were to land at Southampton and all arrangements were made to that effect, thus the delay. We had a beautiful trip over. Time and space does not allow me to detail a thousandth of the beauty of this part of Devonshire or the welcome of the people which is something astounding. They simply overwhelm one with their attention. The kids crawl over you and the girls escort you, arm in arm. Any volunteer who ever enters England will conduct himself more courteously and fight with ten times more spirit with the thoughts of home and such a "mother country." The tales of the Belgium refugees makes one long for the chance to get nearer to the front to help do his small part in a just cause. If our chance comes, I hope we will do our part. Sunday evening a crowd of wounded British went through the streets—they must have forgot their wounds with the ovation they received.

E. A. Poole 17th Battalion N.S. Overseas Forces

The enthusiasm of the autumn of 1914 is well captured in Eugene's letter. However, he, like the rest of the green, untried Canadian Contingent, would have to wait and train for months before crossing to Flanders and France. Retribution for the wrongs inflicted by the invading German forces upon the Belgian refugees would have to be deferred until then. In early November, he writes a quick note to his eldest sister mentioning a visit to an English aunt's and enclosing two items he had sent home.

November 8

Dear Vera,

I received your letter safely this morning. I am visiting my aunt Mrs A. B. Olsen at Waterham. It is a beautiful place as is all of England that I have seen. I have got to be back to base by reveille Monday morning. If you cannot wear this tie give it to one of my friends who can. Did you receive the pillow top safely? Do not let them soak you too much duty.

Lovingly yours, E. A. Poole

In the autumn of 1914, the Canadians moved to Bulford Camp, Salisbury Plain. And then it rained. It rained steadily for weeks. At first, the Canadians lived in tents. By December, Eugene could report to his mother that they were in huts. Over thirty thousand troops living, marching, and training on grassy fields in the rain soon turned the scene into a muddy quagmire. Luckily, Eugene's monotony was relieved by a short period of leave: four days away from the mud and rain with the added benefit of relatives to visit—Aunt Mary and her husband Dr Olsen.

December 8
Bulford Camp, England
Dear Mother,

I just received your letter, or Ida's to be exact, and judge by it that the letter I wrote to father could not have reached home because I asked for a few 69th badges and there was no mention of them. Perhaps you know that we are a kilted regiment. When the 69th detachment joined into the N. S. Highlanders [17th Battalion] I had to take down a stripe but there may be opportunities in the future to get it back. I spent a four days leave in London and Waterham. Aunty Mary is just 17 miles by the posts from Westminster Bridge. I had an enjoyable time while there. Dr Olsen and she are fine; the children are well mannered to a degree that is surprising—the two boys go to private school which is very expensive. They are 7th Day Adventists and vegetarians, that is, the whole family. We are living now in huts about 18 ft by 60 ft about 40 men to a hut. It has rained mostly for the last two months and the mud makes hard ploughing or wading. I want to go out to Waterham again if I can get enough cash together to coincide with a pass. You can figure about how many pounds I receive at the end of the month. Well give my regards to all, with love.

I remain your son E. A. Poole.

1915

Four months elapsed until his next surviving letter home. He admits he has not written but now he has news: he has volunteered to join the cyclists. He did so with the expectation that he would see France sooner. It actually had the opposite effect, as extra training was required. He clearly enjoys his new position even if it necessitated another reduction in both rank and pay. He asks his sister to intervene with his father to send funds to Aunt Mary so that he can have a reserve to draw upon when necessary. As Eugene coyly notes, he has found on his travels that wherever he is money seems to be necessary.

April 10
Shorncliffe Camp, England

Dear Sis,

As you see by this letter I am still in England altho in full sight of France. I have not written lately as I fully expected to have been in France by this time as a lot of Nova Scotians are, but we have been held as a reserve and only been picked as drafts when needed and I have not yet been called. You will be surprised to hear I am now a cyclist! They asked for volunteers for the "divisional cycle corp" and I, thinking that it would mean seeing the front sooner, have got on it. We will be in Hounslow 12 miles from London for a short time and then for some merry sport. My accomplishments will be, and in fact are now, expert cyclist, motor cycle, signaling "Morse code" etc. Some study and work I've had to do. We will have none of the hardships of the trenches but will have lots of chances for 'distinction or extinction' all right.

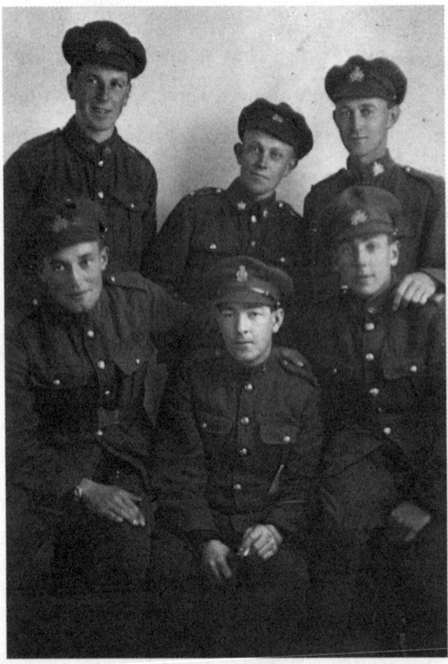

Eugene (top right standing) with five young chums. Notice the large "cyclist" cap badges on five of the men.

Some of my friends will be pleased to know that Lt De V. Chipman is our officer. Your interpretation of CCCF with which I signed off my last letter was correct tho somewhat silly of you not to have known it. If I had come to England on a pleasure trip we could not have found a more appropriate place than Folkstone, a summer resort nearby where we are. The weather here is very spring like and our quarters are fine. The Lark Hill mud is beginning to be a dream of the past. If you get this letter in any kind of season please write and ask father if he can spare a few pounds to send Aunt Mary as I can then draw some from her as I will. No matter where I may happen to be and anywhere I have been yet, money has been of some use. My allowance of pay is pretty small and irregular at that, so thus the plea for a relief fund. I got your last OK and the snaps. I have not written because I wanted my letter to bear the "active service stamp" when next they arrived. Hope you will like the souvenir enclosed. Would have sent more only did not have change enough to get them. Send my best wishes to all home and remember me to all my friends. If any one wonders why I am not in the trenches tell them that the opportunity is still strong for seeing all the fighting one needs.

Yours lovingly Corp E.A. Poole

PS: I reverted again when I volunteered. It takes me most of the time changing stripes.

Eugene finally gets around to writing his mother again. Unabashed and undeterred, he does not hesitate in the least to brag of his accomplishments as a cyclist and of the awaiting dangers—and all this to his mother! He tells her of his pay difficulties, of being in hospital with the measles and of the wonderful heroic and bloody stand the Canadians made against the first ever poison gas attack at the Second Battle Ypres.

May 23

Dear Mother,

It is some time since I have written home so no doubt you will be pleased to hear from me if this letter survives the passage across. There will be a few weeks before we will see France yet but as the cyclists are even ahead of the outposts at the front, then at the rear of the machine guns in a retreat, there is still plenty of time for Victoria Crosses or DCM's yet. If I don't get a commission soon I will have so many decorations to wear that my sleeve won't hold them all. Marksman's crossed rifle, musketry instructor's badge above my stripes, signalling flags and cyclist badge. If I ever live to get back home it will be better than going to a vaudeville show to go to the little volunteer play camps.[3] There is one thing I should have mentioned sooner is regarding my assigned pay home, on secondary consideration I signed 25 cents home and the pay office claims they have sent $40 which placed me $6 or so in debt up to May 1st. May and June will clear me as I stopped it, but it put me in no position to draw money. I went to the hospital for 12 days with German measles and was given 9 days furlough on coming out and no money forthcoming. The best opportunity which I will ever have of seeing merry England at her best and I was forced to resign. A lot of our fellows have been wounded and some killed, but we have done great work and won lots of glory and no man has died in vain. If we don't conquer the Germans there will be no use for our lives anyway. There will be no trouble for the survivors to find a girl in England, they are as thick as black flies are at about this time at home.

3 Eugene's reference to the pre-war summertime militia training camps that some had criticized as little more than male camping socials—an evaluation Eugene now seems to share.

The papers make a great shout over war babies in England. Around here it is a question which are thicker—bicycles or baby carriages. I am only a 6.5 cent ride and return from London, if I ever get a few pounds I will go in and see it properly. Hope this letter finds you well and prosperous. I will close with love to all.

Writing his dad a few days later, he communicates both sobering information and regret. He is in hospital again, the result of a nasty spill from his bicycle. Eugene, of course, downplays the seriousness and wishes he had not cabled home to inform his folks. As for life in England, he feels that he is sufficiently trained to go do his part, the cost of a decent meal is steep, and they have never heard of his favourite Maritime meal: home-made baked beans.

May 29
Hounslow, England

Dear Father,

I received your letter a few days ago and was pleased though I was certainly amused at it. The difference between this country and home is so great that I often forget that I ever lived in old Nova Scotia. When we left Canada they said just wait til you get in England a £ will be a small fortune. Why a dollar bill in Canada will last far longer with me. A decent meal here costs fully 3/6 (three shillings, six pence), the best one can do, but in the first place that is one thing you can't buy in England and no one knows what baked beans are!

I am in hospital again for a few days, the result of a spill off a bicycle, nothing too hurt, just a bump on the hip and my forearm grazed. One comical fellow here is wounded through the throat. He said he saw the bullet coming but did not have time to dodge it. I am sorry that I cabled home, I might have known that everyone would go off their nut! I would write more about my work but I do not believe in spieling on military matters. Divisional cycle training will cover most everything. I have sometimes wished myself that you had come along too, we could of had some wonderful times. Your comical nature would have helped in this damp atmosphere. I don't think I will be here much longer as I am "personally" trained in most all the branches of the service. However, I am more than eager to take my part when it comes, although a larger number than you people at home know anything about certainly will never come back. Before you ask any more questions of Kitchener[4] take a tip and study up the ammunition! I love the army and if I get through the war will make it my profession.

Love to all, your son E A Poole

Unfortunately for Eugene, his little forearm complaint was not as minor as he first thought, and he was still in hospital convalescing in late August. He covers up his long silence with bravado and questions about the portion of his pay that was assigned to home. On a more serious note, he comments on British wartime attitudes toward men not in uniform and of what he understands to be the true state of those reported as "missing." It is unlikely that such sentiments eased his parents' anxieties.

4 British Empire forces were short of artillery shells, and Lord Kitchener was held to blame.

August 29
Canadian Reserve Cyclist Company,
Hounslow, England

Dear Parents,

How are you all after this long lapse? Worrying the flesh away from you over me I suppose. I am still alive and in good health although banged about some. Have you been watching for my name for a Victoria Cross? It has not arrived yet. One of our chaps has just received the Order of St George from the Tsar, he carried a message under heavy fire up to the first line trench.

There is one thing that worries me; did you received $40.00 assigned pay up until April 1st? The pay office claimed you did which made me about 12£ in debt up to the last of May. If you did you were very foolish not to have sent me some occasionally then I would never have had to enquire into it. If you received $25, then let me know by a definite official statement, and there will be some assets due alright. I hope you have gotten by alright. I have often worried over you. Well we'll let it drop. One might as well be in prison as in hospital although we get lots of motor rides and parties, but it's no place for a restless man.

Tomorrow I go to Woolwich to have my arm X-ray photo-ed again. A good trip that will go too quickly. I have never seen or heard of Arthur Whitman[5] either in England or France although he may be pushing up daisies by this time. Lots of our Nova Scotians are, the poor chaps.

In my last letter I forgot to comment on Ethel Saunders marriage which news I received about five weeks ago. It was quite a surprise to me. Over here no girl would dream of associating with, much less marrying a man unless he was in Karkie. If I survive this war of nations I shall marry an English girl you can bank on that; they are true blue. Still I rather want to return single, the thoughts of one or two are quite agreeable.

5 Arthur Whitman (50826), born 1892 in Bridgetown, Nova Scotia; joined at Halifax in March 1915.

Before I close just let me give you a tip; if you ever see me a *missing*[6]—why put on mourning (clothes) because usually there is only a button or so left to pick up for a souvenir. Anyway, I have 9 lives and am coming home whole or about so. Please don't think me heartless but it's useless being serious—must ring off. As I have said before do not ever worry over me. Yours with love to all and remember me to all my friends.

1916

On March 24, 1916, Eugene's unit, 3rd Canadian Division Cyclists, left England for the continent. On the 30th, they reached a small village called Poperinghe, just outside Ypres, Belgium. There, as part of the British Empire's forces on the Western Front, they got to work. Duties included the mundane such as sentry duty and assisting the military police with traffic control to more rigorous activities such as bridge building and dugout construction. The latter two activities were of great interest to the Germans and were often carried out under enemy shellfire. Unfortunately for the Canadians, the entire area was within easy range of massed German artillery.

Eugene writes a very informative letter to his sister Vera. He alternates between home matters and the reality of his daily struggle to survive. He speaks of the mayflowers she promised to send him and he worries about their father being ill and about the impact this will have on family finances. Most touchingly, he offers some brotherly advise on Vera's interest in becoming a nurse. He also tells his sister about the whine of incoming shells, of shrapnel, of "Blighty wounds," muddy roads, and his development of an uncharacteristic lack of interest in dancing.

6 A military casualty classification; others included POW (prisoner of war) and DOW (died of wounds).

April 17
No 3 Platoon, 3rd Canadian Divisional Cyclists, Belgium

Dear Sister,

Don't think Vera that I have forgotten you or anything that memories of you bring back to me, only in my many changes I drift away from the habit of writing as often as I should. My health is good and I am as tough as hard living and lean meat can make me. You should get some photos long before you hear this. My nerves are good too. I often go along where the shrapnel is bursting around and think no more of it than I would of someone snowballing me though I have no cause to love that particular kind of serenade. You hear a whistle in the air before it gets near to you and you commence to wonder where it is going to burst.

The weather here is very changeable, a beautiful warm day then a cold wet one, but we're equipped for all weathers, only the roads are awful to ride in wet weather. We had a snow blockade in England before I left. Something very unusual for England, it snowed for three weeks almost every day, we had some real snow battles too as several black eyes attested.

I am glad that the people of old Novie [Nova Scotia] are commencing to see that it's on this side of the hemisphere that their homes are being defended; some of the home knitted socks that are sent over here should be given to a few of the civies at home because, after exhausting every excuse, it's a case of cold feet when all is said.

The thing that concerns me most though is father. I can't imagine him being sick. I hope that things aren't tied up too bad financially because I could have three or four pounds coming into the family plate. You perhaps know that the government holds half of our pay in banks in Canada to be paid over at the end of the war or to the person our will is made out to in the event of our "depot." Perhaps I had better make an assignment though to help along. Let me know though how we float. We just get enough here to keep us in fun money here.

A person has to learn to drink beer and coffee here as the water is terrible. The thing that everyone looks forward to is leave to England or going to "Blighty," which is Tommie's idea of getting a wound which is not very serious.

I think kid it's useless for you to be set on being a Red Cross nurse or a nurse at all. You have successfully passed into your present position and think of the long time you would studying and working for your diploma again. Life is too short for one to always be doing it (studying), besides you'll be meeting some Methodist minister with spectacles and a bald head soon and be getting married. Still, without joking, in the interests of patriotism, it would do no harm to write to Captain Clutten stating your inclination and adaptabilities, perhaps a word from him might help you. I can quite understand your feelings in the matter but am not in a position to assist you much.

I am glad to hear about Leila, I had forgotten that she was growing up. I will not know her nor Sport [the family dog] either when I come back.

Dancing don't have the attraction for me it used to. I wouldn't walk across the street to the best ball in the season now. I used to roller-skate in England

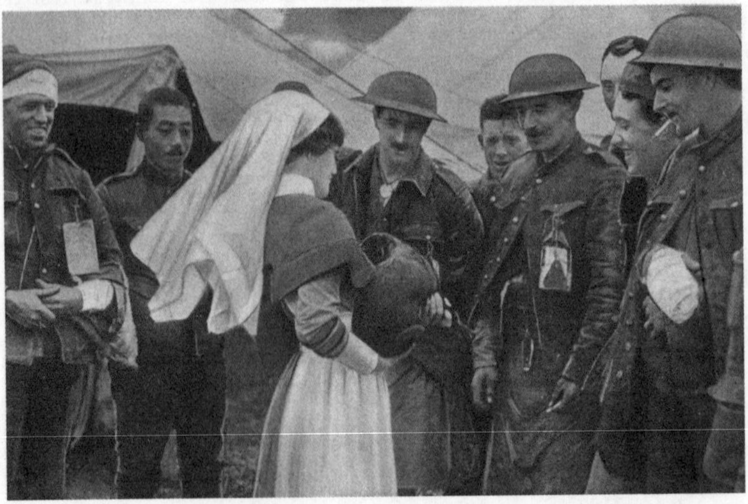

A nursing sister being presented with a dog by wounded Canadian soldiers.

in lieu of ice, how I would liked to have torn up a good smooth piece of honest to god ice though! About the mayflowers, I would appreciate them but you did not reckon on them being June bugs when they got to me, did you? Send me a good old Blue nose Bridgetown paper and I'll be quite satisfied to read that Mr Jones lost a colt of wonderful or doubtful value.

At the time of writing, I am in a Y.M.C.A. camp behind the lines and a merry evening of song, band etc is being carried on, so if some of it gets in here don't blame me as some of the songs are laughable. Fortunately, I had a few hours to read your book [letter] in, don't get a shock when you receive this, I am sure it is more than I have written in the last three months altogether. I must get down the line now and see how much sleep is coming to me. We go to bed here with the hens or as the owl, but mostly when we have the opportunity. I am sending you a few photos to keep for me as I may lose them.

With love from your brother. E. A. Poole

A few days later Eugene writes his dad. Although he is clearly in the thick of things, with booming artillery, chums getting roughed up, and the anniversary of the German gas attack, Eugene's thoughts are of home. He says news that his dad has been ill worries him more than all the German artillery. He wonders if his dog will still know him upon his return, and he craves a pound of "real" Nova Scotia homemade butter! Finally, he announces that he will assign even more of his pay to home to help out the family finances.

April 22
Belgium

Dear Father,

Received a letter from Vera lately and she mentioned that you were sick with the pleurisy. I hope to hear soon that you are yourself again. It seems so strange for the old iron horse to go wrong that it worries me more than any of Fritz's favourite shells. The weather here is simply rotten, it only clears up to rain and it doesn't have to mark time long for that either. Has my dog grown up to be a fool or what is he like? I look forward to seeing him as much as I do anything else nearly. I wonder if he will know me.

Let me know what regiment Arthur Whitman is in or if he is in hospital or wounded, killed or what. It's strange that I have never seen him as almost every fellow I ever knew I have seen over here but never one that knew his name even. Starrett has a staff job where he is safe as if he were home by the fireside, his people need have no fear of him never coming back. Probably it is bad everywhere now though so we will have to make the best of it.

The guns shake things up pretty well around here whether it's wet or dry. My powers of description are limited as to military matters but I will have enough to say when I come back to make up for it all. Four of our fellows got scratched up a bit lately—nothing very serious though. Today is the anniversary of the Germans' first gas attack and the guns boom oftener from our front; the morale of the Canadians has not diminished a particle, rather increased since that time and the gas or other barbarous stratagems have no effect now.

I am billet orderly today so have it pretty soft for a day, thus the inspiration to write a few words. While I think of it, if you are ever anxious to send me anything, send the "Monitor" once in a while or as a special treat send a pound of honest to God butter. It would only be enough for one piece of bread, but I have forgotten what it tastes like. My address is the same as time of last writing so remember it as you will never see it again on any letter. By the way, I think I will get a few pounds assigned home to help the finances.

So long, with love to all, from your son EA Poole

Two weeks later, he writes his youngest sister, Leila. He comments on the lack of correspondence from her, while at the same time sending her some flowers picked on the edge of a large bomb crater. He tells her of a near escape from a shell blast and of his being back at headquarters for a few days' rest. It appears his superiors thought his close call was closer than he lets on to his sister.

May 7
Belgium

Dear Leila,

I don't hear from you very often for some reason or other, perhaps it gets tied up somewhere. The last letter I got from Vera said she wasn't writing any news as Ida was writing that night. I don't mind ordinarily, but have been anxious to hear how father is getting along although from Vera's letter I thought he must be convalescent by the tone of it.

Spring has visited us here and the country around is very pretty—although showing the ravages of shell fire. It is not bad even when we have to sleep out in the open even. Although it's not pleasant on a wet night but we are thankful if we have a sandbag at our head.

There is absolutely no doubt as to the outcome of the war and I am planning to eat my xmas dinner at home. I had to go through a section under heavy bombardment the other day and it made me jump dodging the shells, one struck on one side of the road while I was lying on the other—the shock nearly paralyzed me and I had a headache for several days, the dust and dirt covered me but the fragments went over me as I was lying down. Of course this sounds wild, but it's quite simple for one used to shell fire to dodge them by the shriek they make coming. The forget me knots (enclosed in the letter to his sister) were picked on the edge of a crater made by a Jack Johnson[7] you could bury a church in.

I am back at our headquarters now having a few days rest before going on duties again. I would rather be on outposts as we eat better there than we do back here and live more regimentally. There isn't much that I can write about out here, you know, if you expect to receive it. I just like to send you a line to let you know that I exist.

Love to all, E. A. Poole

Clearly in the middle of a prolonged period of action, Eugene writes his dad. Living in rain, mud, and constant shellfire, he forces himself to write home on a regular basis. It is his connection to the world and the life he once knew. Eugene's sense of humour and knowledge of rural life shines through in the comment to his dad to ensure that his mother should not open an enclosed letter "by accident or curiosity."

7 The nickname given to a very large German explosive shell.

May 15
Flanders, Belgium

Dear Father,

I received the last family budget recently and was glad to hear that you are getting around again. While I think of it, I might say that I never heard tell of the post card which Ida was supposed to have sent me, also no card ever arrived from Aunt Bert. I presume she had some silly address on it. Nevertheless, I will drop her a line on the strength of it. I am very sorry that I did not get assigned pay started long ago but you know I had to stop it to get straightened up in finances myself. Since last year they have held back half of the Expedition men's pay except in cases where they have assigned pay. Of course, it will be handy after the war, so if anything should happen to me, don't forget what the government owes you.

There is nothing that I can talk about as you know you can tell where we are though by any newspaper if you have a map and half sense. I am going out on outpost duty tonight and it is a dirty night, still I must be thankful if I have a sandbag between me and Fritz, let alone worrying over the atmospheric conditions. I am pretty well equipped for mud and rain.

It was a great surprise to me to hear of aunt Alma's acquisition, I don't blame her for ceasing to be careful at her time of life, still it's very silly of her. I'll bet Olive is sore. A kid hasn't any business butting in on a settled household. I am sending a note of condolence, if you can call it that, to Ethel Saunders, or at least the Ethel I knew. Please send it along to its destination and don't let mother open it by mistake or curiosity. I wish I could send some of the curios home that I get hold of at times but it's impossible. Well I haven't said much but just promised myself that I would try and write regular whether I wrote anything of news of not.

Love to all, your son EA Poole.

The shellfire in the Ypres area continued to be intense. Eugene writes his sister Vera at the end of May commenting that "it's very warm out here now literally and figuratively." Being "warm" was army slang for a very dangerous place. At this point in the war, the unit's war diary indicates Eugene's cyclists were assigned to assist the engineers in the construction of water lines to supply suitable bathing and drinking water for the tens of thousands of troops in the vicinity. This no doubt raised his desire to "swim in the old Annapolis river."

Eugene often attempted to lighten the tone of his letters by commenting on news from home and by describing his off-duty activities. In this letter, for instance, he comments on playing baseball and of an unexpected addition to his aunt's family. However, he also admits to not writing a return letter to his sister's friend and of dodging shellfire. Indeed, he is actually under so much stress at this time that he puts the wrong year on the letter.

May 29
Flanders, Belgium

Dear Sister Vera,

I received your long letter not very long ago, I have written home since but not to you. It is very warm out here now literally and figuratively. This weather makes one long for a swim in the old Annapolis river; good baths are provided here behind the lines, but any of the ponds are no better than cess pools filled with leeches as big as an eel. We have quite a lot of fun when not on duty, playing ball, pitching quoits and boxing and for a variety always the whistling of a shell for amusing yourself to see how close the anti-aircraft shells are coming to a plane, often times the pieces of shell from them drop around like rain. But common shell fire does not worry me any. It's when one whistles right over and lights nearby that my blood gets cold for a minute. They say that a shell has to have your number on it to get you, however I'm quite content to get in a ditch when one comes.

Do you know Vera that I never answered the letter that your chum sent me from Truro Normal [school]? It was very rude of me as it was particularly nice, but if you will give me her address and pave the way for me with an apology, I will try and send her a few words.

I was greatly surprised to hear of aunt Alma's addition. I will take great pleasure in eating a goose neck in honour of it when I visit her. Is Viola still teaching school? I haven't heard from her for some time. I answered her letter too. I was glad to get Jesse's note—it sounded very natural. I think you mentioned Carl joining up to something or other didn't you? It was funny about Robert Cameron and his father. Just remember me to any of your friends that happen to know me and cheer up because they say the first seven years will be the worst."

Yours with love, E. A. Poole

The strain of his situation continued to wear on Eugene. The battle of Mount Sorrell was raging, and casualties were high. As for war news, there was a great difference between what the men at the front thought and what their families at home were reading in the papers. Eugene characterizes some of what he reads from recruiting bulletins and Canadian newspapers as nothing short of "ridiculous." All the while the shells continued to fall.

June 9
Flanders, Belgium

Dearest Sister,

I received your letter "book" not many days ago and the parcel yesterday. It could not have been more appropriate if you had asked my choice. By the time you receive this you will just about be getting ready for your vacation. I should judge and I hope that you will have a good time too. The news from home was very interesting but some of the new battalions recruiting bulletins and the newspapers war news are nothing short of ridiculous, although I expect the people home look on them with real seriousness. I should like to see father's namesake who I see is in training in some glorious regiment, I forget the number (seven hundred and some odd figures, I think) when a shell goes by him. I'll bet the next one wouldn't. There have been some awful offences on both sides lately. I guess some of the fellows who go back to Canada will not consider Hell an awful thing to look forward to.

I expect to be going back for a rest shortly. It mostly means cleaner dress buttons, badges and boots. If they don't improve the opportunity to teach something that we are beginning to forget, I'll have no kick. You should hear a shell coming over as big as a hogshead, they sound like an express train coming along. Of course, they don't commonly snipe at you with these little souvenirs but you never know when a bombardment is going to commence. At present it is in the form of huge raincoats and me 3/4 of an hour from my billet with no raincoat.

I wrote a letter to Viola not long ago. I talked to her as if she was a little kid. I just remembered afterward that she is pretty well grown up. Tell Jesse that I appreciated his note very much

People in England say that the war will finish in August; out here they say the first seven years will be the worst; so work it out algebraically if you wish. Well, don't take all this too seriously, my sense of humour is rather crude.

Yours with love, E. A. Poole

Humour was an essential survival strategy. The English soldier Bruce Bairnsfather's humorous sketches of life in France and Flanders became famous during the war. Eugene also mentions his father's sense of humour and attempts some humour himself. Regarding his emotional health, he references his "nerves"—that is, if he had any left! In this instance, the dark humour is rather appropriate, as it appears he was in a forward area for another eight-day stint. His strained nerves are apparent with his very curt words to his father about publishing any more of his letters home in the local newspaper.

July 6
Belgium
Dear Father,

It is encouraging to hear from you again. Your sense of humour will always keep you alive. It was rotten that you were taken sick just as you were and it's too bad that with all the money I have to my credit in London, I am not able to get at it here to help you make up for the lost time. When I go on leave to London again I will spend less and send home a roll. The weather conditions have been good lately and Fritz has been quite tame. Also in this part for a change, several bombs were dropped nearby yesterday without much damage being done. One of them fell quite close to where I was. I am afraid that they would dent my helmet if they fell on it.

9/7/1916 I was obliged to quit here and this is the first chance to resume writing. I got Vera's letter last night and the one from home before Vera's. It was very amusing that you thought my birthday to be on the 10th of June. Your little holiday trip must have taken some planning to carry out successfully, it was worthy of a general. I came up here this morning and will be here for eight days if all goes well. By the way, lest I forget to mention it, don't stick anymore of my letters in the paper and then have the nerve to send me one. When I want one published I will let you know. Some people think the war will be over soon, I think so too now that Frank Poole jr has enlisted for overseas. I have been quite a long while answering letters but have been very busy lately so excuse this rambling letter. It's is the best that I can do. It must be lovely home now, the weather has been fairly good here even for some time. One fellow wrote home that the weather conditions continued very steady, will send a wire when the rain stops.

I like the little notes I get from mother. Simplicity is Truth. I did not know that Leila was so interested in flowers or I could have sent lots of them. I will send one in this letter though the pressing may be amateur. I will send this letter out at first opportunity, pardon the jerkiness of it, although my nerves are very good if I've got any. Do you ever see any of the Bairnsfather fragments from Flanders? They are simply wonderful and vetoed by all soldiers. I hope this finds you all well as this leaves me.

Love to all, your son E. A. Poole

Eugene's next letter to his father is very revealing of his altered mental state. He mentions his state of mind several times, and admits that he is uncharacteristically short on words to write. He tells his father, only half-jokingly, to write their MP, J. E. Morse, and ask about a commission as an officer in one of the newly formed battalions back in Canada. Next, he muses about leaving the Canadians for the British army—whatever it takes to escape his present situation, which appeared increasingly hopeless. All this is stated against the background of the experience of a family acquaintance, Harry Starrett, who was one of only four out of a group of eighteen who escaped death when a six-inch German shell landed in their midst. Undoubtedly, Eugene had seen repeated instances of such unpredictable and indiscriminate death by shell fire.

August 30
Flanders

Dear Father,

I received your last letter but have not received the parcel or papers yet. To tell you the truth I don't know my address yet but call it Canadian Corps Cyclist c/o Camp Commandant 4th Division until I am better informed. I expect I am on the sub-staff. I have not been in a very good position to write for sometime but do not be surprised at any address I may give you in the future. But do not expect me home for that xmas dinner this year.

I saw H. Starrett not long ago. He is the same Harry. He has been very lucky, one of only four who were left from a party of eighteen who were an obstacle in the path of a German 6 inch shell.

The weather has been good lately but it seems to have changed the last few days so now we can expect it wet for a while. The wind and rain today seems to have a touch of fall in it and the winter is not a pleasing thought but we should not worry. I wish you would write J. E. Morse and ask him how chances are to get a commission in some battalion in Canada who are likely to be coming overseas at an early date. It would be quite simple if he would give me a chance.

The news is of a necessity dull from me and I have been away from home so long that my mind is blank. The letters from the girls are a great help to me to keep me from getting quite stale, but my mind is bent on a change and if J. E. does nothing I will get into the English army much as I hate to lose my identity with the Canadians. It will be very nice having Vera home this year or so near home though Ida will be away perhaps. What seems to be the opinion of the war at home? I am always interested to hear although it's often a matter for merriment for me. Will write more fully in next letter but I am poor in vocabulary today.

Your son, with love, E. A. Poole

A few weeks later matters seem improved, as Eugene writes his mother asking her to send him a little money in case he secures some leave.

September 12

Dear Mother,

This date finds me in the best of health as usual. I am just writing business (in this note) this morning so don't get startled. On receipt of a certain money order which will arrive to you or your name please deduct one £ and hasten it on to me. I don't usually need much money but that much will be acceptable. I am looking forward to leave some time in the far future but it's still out of sight.

Love to all E. A. Poole.
PS: The £ has nothing to do with leave, ha

The steady flow of letters from Nova Scotia meant that thoughts of home were never far from Eugene's mind. He pens a very newsy letter to his sister Vera offering all sorts of brotherly advice to her as she com-

mences teaching school in a nearby village. Eugene's reference to "whizz-bangs" was the soldiers' nickname for a standardized army Field Post Card—the original form letter. It was prewritten, and the soldier simply highlighted what he wanted to say and crossed out what did not apply. They were named after a small-sized German trench mortar round that arrived with little warning.

September 19

Dear Sister Vera,

I can never hope to write enough to meet the letters I get from home, half way even, if it was not for the fact that I enjoy getting correspondence to such an extent I would never send anything, but "Whizz-bangs" (field post cards)—they [the authorities] have the proper [measure] of a letter from a man on active service down fine.

It is great that you are going to be home this year or nearly so at least. Do you know I can't realize having two such learned sisters and another one studying to work. Although I strongly expect she missed her "D" owing to so much puttering over botany. I myself can remember such terms as Oderferus Odsura, Rhododendron Rhodora and can distinguish between calyx and corolla pistil and stamens etc. Oh yes and a lot more when I come to look back. I am glad that you took in the trip to Aldershot, perhaps you know Myra Marshall. We keep up a sort of desultory correspondence. She and Mabel hired a car and she dilated on their trip in a letter which I got not long ago. If she does not go to the Seminary this year you may see her around town and I suggest that you speak to her. Anyway I expect you know her though better than I.

During the winter months I would stay down through the week anyway, it would be too much trying to make it every day, besides you might slide over to the rink occasionally. I sincerely hope that father will manage to make the trip to the exhibition, it's too bad that he has to work so hard after the sickness he went through. Although his light heartedness and sense of humour will take him anywhere. It makes my mouth water to hear blueberry pie mentioned. It's been over two years now since I have had anything that could really be called a pie—although for active service food we have no kick whatever in the way we live. I think I have mentioned that it chiefly clears up to allow it to rain some more and the soil being naturally wet and of clay loam about three fine days are required to dry it, so work out the ratio; wettest, wetter, and wet.

It's always a treat to hear from mother; one gets well supplied with inside information. You will have received some mail by this time. I expect it seems that I have written oftener than you mention though. Oh, by the way, the two brothers you asked about are named Andrews, A.P. and A.E., they used to be in my platoon, fine boys too. Quite a number of the chaps in the large picture have been killed and wounded and big changes have occurred since the time that picture was taken. I will close and just add that APM means Army Provost Marshall and APO Army Post Office. Anyway you have my address by now.

With love to all E. A. Poole

In mid-September 1916, the Canadian troops were thrown into the ongoing Battle of the Somme. The struggle for the town of Courcelette was a very bloody affair. Along with infantry battalions from across Canada, the two Maritime Battalions, the 25th of Nova Scotia and the Fighting 26th of New Brunswick, suffered significant casualties. During the battle, members of the cyclist battalion carried ammunition, food, and especially water forward at night—under artillery fire. They returned carrying the wounded on stretchers and escorting German prisoners to the POW cages behind the lines. These events are reflected and revealed in Eugene's correspondence by a seven-week silence. His correspondence, now addressed from France instead of the familiar Flanders, resumes in early November. The battle is past. He is still alive and now has time to write home.

November 7
France

Dear Father,

I received your letter a few days ago and was glad to hear from you as it has been some time since I have heard from home. Before I write any further, I would like to have you understand my address. It is Canadian Corps Cyclist Battalion C Company, BEF unless I transfer to something else, the fact that I may be attached at different times to something else, which does not affect it any. After the big offensive we are now on a quiet front, that is to say, we have nothing more exciting than bullets, whiz-bangs, minnie-wavers, trench mortars etc coming over from the Germans. Anyway, they have to be good to get us as they say. The weather is getting pretty bad which, of course, means plenty of mud.

We are living in a dug-out which at one time was a French cellar, the furnishing is rather plain but we have a few frescoed pictures on the wall, it is easy to get to bed but the concrete don't have much spring to it, the rats dispute our claim which no doubt is of a longer standing than ours. I had a rare treat this afternoon—a bath.

How near to the correct time did the birthday card to father arrive? It seems to take longer for mail to reach home than it used to. Still we are lucky to have the service we have. I received the Red Cross parcel not long ago and it was much appreciated. Well I have nothing more to write about and no complaints to make so will get under my blanket.

Your loving son, E. A. Poole
PS: Let me know if you get my remittance.

Being out of the battle area and at rest, Eugene takes the opportunity to write his sisters. He tells Ida that he has had some pictures taken but at an exorbitant price. The men often felt they were being gouged by opportunistic entrepreneurs. Her mention of someone's getting married brings feeling of separation and isolation to the surface, and Eugene muses that all the girls in Canada will have forgotten him by now. Also worthy of note is his comment regarding Sunday as just another day in the week. This was most certainly not how he was raised nor was it the attitude prevalent in Canada at the time. But the war was bringing significant and enduring changes in both attitude and outlook, and religion was certainly not exempt.

November 19
France

Dear Ida,

I have just received your last letter, it was nearly a month old. I presume it went to the reserve in England first, please write my address; Can Corps Cyc Batt C Coy # 3 Platoon, BEF. We are enjoying a week's rest and are making the most of it before we go out again. The xmas souvenirs are very nice and perhaps you may receive a small remembrance from yours truly. The boys I chum with and myself had some pictures taken today. We had to give the photographer enough to keep him over xmas but thought you would all appreciate one. I never knew that Arthur Foster was married but was glad to hear that he was a family man. Don't expect to ever be one myself unless I find a petit French mademoiselle. The girls I used to know in Canada will have forgotten all about me. This is a fine town we are in now. The night before last we went to the theatre, last night to the cinema and tonight being dimanche we will do something equally grand—Sunday being merely one day in the week! The weather has been grand lately but don't know for how long, it's pretty bad in the trenches when it's wet. I received the two pair of socks from the Red Cross, also a check from home not long ago in case I forget to tell them at home when I write. By the time you receive this you will be thinking of the xmas holidays. Will you have a tree this year? I remember Leona White who you mentioned, just give her my best wishes please and good luck for the years work. With so apt a instructor, she should do fine. I am enclosing these stamps. I hope they will be of use. You may wonder how I came by them but no matter.

With best love from your brother, E. A. Poole

Eugene writes his sister Vera the very next day, and it is worth noting the differences between the two letters: no mention of being swindled by the photographer, but he does comment on the quality of the billets they are in and the attitude of the French population. Almost every French family had suffered loss, and they lived life one day at a time, not in prayer, but in seeking out and eking out life's pleasures. Eugene's deep distain for the version of the war found in the newspapers shines through, too. He was especially cynical about what had become the obligatory newspaper reference to the troops' morale. According to the papers, troop morale was always high. Eugene knew first-hand the fluctuations in morale. How could morale be high when so many of your chums were killed, maimed, and missing after a battle? The newspaper accounts were in reality high fiction!

November 20
France

Dear Vera,

Just a few lines to let you know that I received your letter and check OK. I have been back resting for a few days and have made the most of my time. I had some photos taken and will send some shortly. The xmas souvenirs are very nice too and I will try and send a few. There is a theatre nearby and several moving pictures also, so the evenings are very well spent, the place we are billeted in is situated on a hill and is far better than the usual rest billet as is also the village itself. The French people believe in pleasure. Most of the estaminets have a penny-in-the-slot piano and you will see them dancing their legs nearly off. They have had it pretty rou-gh in this war too, few families have not been affected.

The weather has been pretty good lately, in fact very good, real sharp fall weather. I would very much like to get leave sometime now but as lots of fellows are more entitled to it than me, (I'll have to wait)—still one has to hope for something and that's about the only thing to look forward to.

Well the news is not very plentiful at least I don't know what constitutes news but I sometimes see a paper which claims we are winning the war and then comes the obligatory sentiment concerning "the spirit of the troops." It's a great sight to watch our aeroplanes in the air. The English have it all over the Germans in that line. It is a game which appeals to me, but I must be content to fly with one foot on the ground I suppose. Well, scoff is up, so will ring off.
Yours with love.

Eugene even had time to write a letter to his Aunt Mary Olsen in England, whom he had visited earlier at the beginning of the year while on leave. While commenting on the poor weather and the incessant mud, he also mentions that he hopes to visit her on leave sometime in the spring. Eugene has a long wait of wet, cold, mud, and danger ahead of him.

November 27
France

Dear Aunt Mary,

Just a few lines to let you know that I am OK and am having plenty of work and expect to see you about spring, if I don't get a "Blighty" first. I have been a bit worried over the five pounds I remitted you on the 25th October. Please let me know if you received it, if not, I will inform the pay master to that effect. I expect the weather is none to good in England. The mud in the trenches is pretty bad. I hope this finds everybody in good health. I would like to take a walk with the boys, also I would enjoy looking across your dining room table at the present moment.

Remember me to friends at the "Hydro," love to all, E. A. Poole

Given the minimum time lag of at least six weeks between sending a letter and receiving a reply, Eugene's late-November reference to Christmas should come as no surprise. In fact, he penned his Christmas letters home in early December. They are an interesting blend, as he alternates between war-weariness, homesickness, and reassurances to family that he is both safe and in good spirits.

December 7
France

Dear Mother,

This letter should reach you about xmas I think. By this time you will have received my remembrances of the season. You may wonder where I got funds to get them, but the pay was enlarged on last month in order for soldiers to send home souvenirs. I was not able to give everyone an equal show, but hope you will like my choice of presents. The tea apron to Vera was quite a splash, as Laura used to say, "it cost enough." Unless our shift changes, you can think of me on Xmas day enjoying myself as best as possible somewhere in the "trenches" or near them anyway. Don't think that I shall be miserable though because I shall be feeling cheerful enough—nothing like being optimistic! One gets used to everything out here, besides I am looking forward to leave at an early date.

Did you think I looked all right in my photo? Except for being rather thin I am in first class condition. The photographer was not anything wonderful of course, but I know you always like to see my picture from time to time. Ida said you liked the Bairnsfather drawing, the best of them, they are very true to real life at the front and are more appreciated by men who have seen the same conditions. Our xmas cards have not arrived yet but I will send one along when they arrive. They will be something like last years, only have the Corps colours instead of the 1st Division blue.

I was glad to get the papers from home and I noticed some of the local casualties were published but not all, as I know quite well. Harry Starrett is an officer in B Coy cyclists. "Joe" has not changed much since you knew him last, nothing could ever make him much different.

It makes me a little sore sometimes to read of the boys around home that never had any idea of the army holding commissions—imagine little

Ralph Layte[8] being Capt and Adj even though the battalion has three numbers in it and will never reach France as a unit. Still I wish them all luck and honours. DeBlois Anderson[9] won his commission on the field out here and if ever a man deserved it 'twas him; he was the most popular NCO in his battalion.

Well this is not a very cheerful letter to write home but I am really feeling thankful that I am as I am and wish for nothing better. I want you to collect up my certificates of education; musketry, certificate of rank etc., in active militia, get a recommendation from Col McNeil or Major Morse and also a note of moral standing from the minister as to my moral standing, perhaps a note from the mayor. Don't get alarmed at all by this but if you collect this bunch send them to aunt Mary's in England as I may wish to start something if I get on leave, if not, no harm will be done.

Are you going to have the usual xmas tree this year? I don't think I will hang up my stocking this year, as the rats would probably take it to line their winter quarters with. I heard from Ida the other day and expect I will hear from home tonight maybe. Everything is OK and "the spirits of the troops are excellent," with love to all. your loving son E. A. Poole

A few days later, at the front and down deep in a dugout, Eugene pens his sister a Christmas letter. As well as mentioning the fact that the official battalion Christmas cards had not yet been handed out, he also speaks of rats, snow, and the full moon. The last item is a particular worry to someone whose work was mostly at night, under the cover of darkness, with the hope of remaining unseen by the enemy.

8 Lieutenant Ralph R. Layte, born Boston, 1893, living in Paradise, Nova Scotia, and also a former member of the 69th Militia Regimen

9 Lieutenant DeBlois Anderson, born Dalhousie, Ann County, Nova Scotia, 1893, and also a former member of the 69th Militia Regiment.

December 11
France

Dear Sister,

I will improve the few minutes before dinner writing to you as are most of the boys in the dugout writing or reading. I arrived in late last night so I am still between the blankets. The day is beautiful outside and the aeroplanes are making good use of it. The moon is full in the sky now so when it is not misty one is very nervous on top at night, quite as bad as when the star shells explode. I was surprised to hear that snow stayed so long in November at home. We haven't had any yet to speak of, about February is the snowball season here.

The weather has been disagreeable lately but as usual the worst is yet to come. I have felt pretty good all along, only a slight cold in all. We have a pretty good billet but it's got nothing on our cellar except our old friends the rats. Your parcel has not arrived yet but there is lots of time. The address will be rather weird though if it was the same as the letters. The xmas cards have not been given out yet so if you receive a greetings of the season card for Easter with mistletoe wreath on them, why refer back to 25/12/16. I expect to get leave some time the first of the year. I will try and remember you all when that event happens. I think uncle Mayor must have meant that aunt Mary had been visiting him last summer. Surely she is not over again. Well, "scoff" is about up and it's time I was too.

Yours as B4 in bed, E. A. Poole

On Christmas night Eugene writes a letter to his mother describing his last twenty-four hours. By 1916 there was no longer any appetite on either side for a truce. Eugene did admit that Christmas Eve had been somewhat quieter with respect to artillery, but besides that the only indication of Christmas was a sign in the officers' dugout and a "pretty good

Christmas dinner." As he got dressed to go out on Christmas night, the guns were at it again, and he sarcastically notes the end of the "Day of Peace."

December 25,
France

Dear Mother,

Just a few lines on Xmas night to give you some idea of how we spent the day. On xmas eve we went out all night on a working party but the line was pretty quiet, both sides remembering the date although nothing much different was noticed except the sign in the officers dugout "Merry Xmas to All." Most of the day was spent in sleeping but tonight for high tea we had a pretty good xmas dinner consisting of mashed potatoes, cabbage, chicken, pudding, cake, oranges and nuts.

Besides numerous parcels which were received by the boys in our dugout I got your parcel safely and it was much appreciated. I also received another from Washington D.C.—a very fine one. Well, I haven't much to say. I hope that my presents reached you in time for xmas and that you all had a good day. I expect to get on leave some time before long. I will have my time then. I must get dressed now to go out shortly. It is just one damn thing after another as the saying goes. I guess the "day of Peace" is over by the sound of the guns, however, we should worry.

With love to all E. A. Poole

1917

In the winter of 1917, all four divisions of the Canadian forces serving on the Western Front were brought together for the first time. Their orders were to attack, capture, and hold an area of high ground in France known as Vimy Ridge. In January and February, the Cyclists' War Diary states that they were working with the tunnelling companies for weeks on end. This involved construction of the miles of tunnels leading to the battlefield. It was within these miles of tunnels that the Canadian infantry safely advanced and then waited for the battle to begin. During the battle, many cyclists were detailed to escort captured prisoners to the rear—a dangerous task while under shellfire. Other cyclists were attached to various infantry battalions as newly created specialized Lewis machine-gun crews to augment the fire power of the attacking units. On Easter Monday, April 9, 1917, the one-hundred-thousand-strong Canadian Corps under the command of British general Julian Byng launched its attack. After several days of bloody fighting, the Canadians took and held the ridge. This was the greatest Allied victory of the war thus far. Newspapers throughout the Empire and in France heralded the victory. But even victory in the Great War was very costly: 3,500 Canadians died taking and holding Vimy Ridge and more than twice that number were wounded. After a long gap in correspondence, Eugene writes his mother at the end of April.

April 27
France

Dear Mother,

I received your letter some few days ago, also the papers, both of which were appreciated. I particularly like to get a letter from you. I always know how everything stands at home. Both of the girls have written but I am very slow in writing, it is very difficult to concentrate my mind on any subject to write about. It may interest you to know that I have secured a small monthly assignment which may come in handy as at present the prices of living must be a tax on economy. The flowers I am sending I have carried in my pay book for some time. They grew near a famous old church tower which has sentinelled[10] more than one bloody battle. The present advance which is being carried on now is terrific—it's a wonderful thing to see the panorama viewed from the ridges wrestled from Fritz. I am glad that everyone is in good health at home and hope that father has tried to go easy this spring. Don't let him over tax himself too much after a sickness like his. He wants to be careful. I want the family complete when I get back; I haven't acquired much honour or glory, nor have I grasped my opportunities but the war is still young yet so there is still time. I was sorry to hear of Hilda B's death, if you have the opportunity please convey my sincere regrets for one of my oldest schoolmates to Mr and Mrs A. Daniels, also to Frank B. The weather still continues cold but spring will soon be here I think now. Well, so long for the present. Love to all.

Yours lovingly, E. A. Poole

Eugene's reference to honour and glory is, of course, an ironic one. By this stage of the war, he had seen much maiming and death, but he cannot, and most definitely will not, tell his family the gruesome truth. And so this irony is his outlet. Eugene has come to the realization that his major challenge is not to garner glory but to stay alive—to live to fight another day and, he hopes, some day to return home. When writing to his sister a month later, his war-weariness and sense that any leave is a forlorn hope comes through very clearly. So too does the danger he is in, for he writes from a dugout whose ceiling is constantly dropping dirt on his letter due to an ongoing German bombardment.

10 Eugene's reference is most likely to the famous cathedral in Albert, France.

May 21
France

Dear Sister,

I received all your letters some few days ago. I don't write very often chiefly because I have nothing to write about. It doesn't pay to shoot a heavy line—I might see it in the paper again. I get pretty tired and fed up after we have been in one place for long; while we are moving it is not so bad; it is the steady grind of the same front that gets one. We are living in what was recently a German dugout in a town captured from them. At present he is dropping stuff around pretty close, in other words, I am writing under shell fire. On the door the sign reads Vorsicht Gargefahr which means beware of gas. The room is all nicely papered etc. Fritz always believes in comfort wherever he is. The weather has been good for about a month now but April was very wintry for the most part, but spring has made a show in places where one would have thought all life was extinct. There are not many of us who are looking for a very speedy outcome of the war, so it will be some time yet before I can get home. I have not heard from Dr Olsen for some time chiefly because I am looking for some money which he has of mine, I presume. Besides, he is always looking for me on leave—what a hope! If you write to Miss Millet again thank her for looking after my letter so well. Maybe I will write myself sometime. I don't write to any girls in Canada. Well you can truthfully say that this letter has been well christened as pieces have been falling the whole time I have been writing. I hope my assignment of pay to home has begun to take effect by this time.

Your loving brother, E. A. Poole

Ten days later, still at the front and down in a dugout, Eugene writes his sister Ida. He answers questions about who he has seen and what he thinks of the war and the new soldiers coming over from Canada. His comments on the life expectancy of reinforcements are very revealing. They can try for a safe position (very unlikely) or hope to get a wound serious enough to send them to England (a Blighty one) or they will end up napoo*—Hindustani for killed. What is most telling, however, is his devil-may-care attitude as a First Contingent man toward all these latecomers.*

May 31
France

Dearest Sister,

I have been a little longer than I meant to be answering your letter but I managed to write to Vera so you know that I am all right. The last letter I got from home was a hum-dinger; I used up nearly all my candle reading it through. I am chiefly interested in the production of your play. I hope that it came off with a full house. It was well advertized at any rate. I was glad to hear of your interest in the use of your money, with my income which I have recently placed at mother's disposal, we should make quite a strong syndicate towards the end you mentioned.

At present I am on a night post job and it's a pretty lonesome vigil. I can assure you though it only lasts a week, then we get another posting, perhaps better but still maybe not so good, though a cinch compared to some. I am feeling pretty cheerful these days with the prospect of the war finishing in about two more years—if the people (at home) economize.[11]

11 Rationing and recycling of metals and other war material was in full swing on the home front by this time. Eugene's comment is a sarcastic one. He knows that only the destruction of the German armies on the Western Front will actually end the war.

Also I see just a dim possibility of getting leave in a month or so, enough to live in hope on anyway.

The fates were against me with this letter as a couple of pages of my rambling tale was reduced to char. This is morning now and it is going to be a lovely day, the weather leaves nothing to be desired of late except it brings a wish for the sea shore. After all the terrific devastation by shelling the green leaves appear on battered trees and the birds sing and the many bright flowers peep out even close to the line. I have never seen any of the boys you mention out here or I think it was Leila who mentioned it. I don't seem to remember them at all. Most of the fellows in an umpty-umpty-ddith[12] Battalion leave England as a draft to some other regiment. They no doubt become the best of soldiers if they are lucky enough to get a blighty [wound] or a bomb-proof [position] before they are napoo [killed]. Still an old 1st Contingent man never forgives them for their tardiness, chiefly because they were not so big a fool as he. Well, sorry I haven't any more time to write now as I must get back and sleep and eat. Remember me to Bertha Corbett if you ever write to her or see her.

Your loving brother, E A Poole

At the end of July, Eugene writes his sister Vera. Although clearly weary and longing for leave, he nonetheless gives his younger sister some brotherly advice regarding her career. The brief note ends with a postscript regarding yet another soldier's death about which his family had informed him.

12 A battalion with a numerical designation over 100.

June 25
France

Dear Sister,

I received your letter some time ago but am just answering it. There is much I could write about—but a whiz-bang describes my sentiments quite well. The weather is too fine to have any old "fed up" feeling even if we only draw enough money in this country to keep cheerfully broke most of the time. I am not surprised to hear you wanting to change your vocation, the business course idea is a good one. You would do well to write Mae Millet at 172 Robie St., Halifax. She could tell you a lot of things and would be glad to do it, so just drop her a line and ask her about the most economical system to go about it. Your education thus far will pass you over the elementary course. Well, by the time you receive this you should be enjoying your vacation and I perhaps will be on leave. Hastily, your loving brother E. A. Poole

PS: I never saw Frank Rice.[13] *I knew him well, though and was sorry to hear he had been killed out here.*

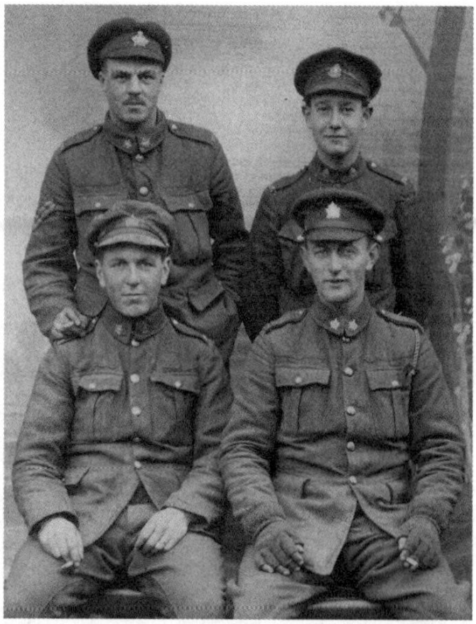

Eugene seated on the right with three chums. Notice his fingertip-less gloves for working with telephone wires.

13 Frank S. Rice (116289), born May 5, 1893, at Deepbrook, Annapolis County, Nova Scotia; killed April 10, 1917.

In July 1917 the battalion was out of the line at Divion and training the new recruits who had arrived from England to replace the men wounded and killed in the recent battles. It was at this period, after approximately a year of waiting, that Eugene's leave finally materialized. He was granted ten days. The relief experienced in leaving the trenches, the shelled zone at the front, and the danger, was immense. Men often had to sleep a great deal at the start of leave in order to recoup from sleep deprivation, but they then spent the remainder of their leave living life to the fullest and doing everything but thinking of the war. Just after his return to France, Eugene again wrote his mother. Returning to war was not easy, as he relates.

July 26
France

Dear Mother,

Since last writing I have been on leave. I had ten wonderful days, I can assure you, though they passed all too quickly. I spent a lot of my time in a bathing suit and a canoe and did not waste much time sleeping either. When I got back there was a letter waiting for me from Ida. Now that I remember it, there has never been any mention of you receiving any of the assignment pay which you should have got since the 1st of April. Please let me know if it has reached you yet. Everything was lovely in Blighty, the weather was good for the most part, though not so warm as it is here. Yesterday we had a very violent thunder storm with large hail stones. I thought by some of the stories [of rationing] that I would starve on leave but quite the contrary. I had plenty to eat alright. It is a lonesome feeling coming back again but a few days will bring everything natural again. I spent my birthday [July 10] in Blighty anyway. Well don't worry over me, I am likely to be all right for a while anyway.

Your loving son E A Poole

Later that summer, Eugene writes home mentioning his job as a linesman, whose responsibilities included locating and repairing broken telephone lines. He failed, however, to mention two relevant details. First, by this stage of the war, all such lines were buried at a minimum depth of six feet to avoid being cut by enemy artillery fire. Second, the repair had to be carried out immediately, while the German artillery barrage continued, often unabated, for hours. He also mentions the parcel he received from his mother, including hand-knitted socks, and he tells her his parcel content preferences for future reference. Eugene even mentions a rare event—a First Contingent man who was so fortunate as to be sent home on three months' leave. Unfortunately, Eugene would not be so lucky.

August 13
In the Field

Dear Mother,

Just a few lines to let you know that I received your parcel a few days after your letter on the 10th and a letter from Ida and Vera before that. I was glad that you got the assignment all right. I was beginning to worry about it. I expect the girls will be teaching by the time this gets home. They appeared to be liking it at Truro pretty well. I hope everything is running smooth at home and that father is not working too hard. I am sorry about Viola. It seems strange that she can't buck up and get better.

I had a good time while on leave. I was not out of Caterham much, but was well looked after while there. Dr Olsen has since gone on a short visit to Ind., U S A. It's fun going on leave but the gang plank is not crowded so bad coming back!

The weather has been pretty rotten lately and my job as telephone linesman and signaller does not wait for fine weather if a shell hits the wire. However, it is pretty good job and I hope that it lasts for a while at least. The chap in the centre of the picture is going on three months leave to Canada. He is one of the original 14th Battalion men and I met him several times at Salisbury Plains (autumn 1914). Well, as usual, I have not much to say but regarding parcels any homemade cake or candy, biscuits, raisins, jam or preserves is my preference. The socks you knit just came in time. I had no change and just came in soaked to the skin and they were waiting.

Will close with love to all, Your son E. A. Poole

In his next letter, Eugene lets it slip that his job was so dangerous that, quite out of character, the army granted an amazing degree of autonomy to the men who braved such risks. As for applying for a three-month furlough to Canada, Eugene offers both an excuse and a self-realization. His excuse is that to do so would involve running the U-boat gauntlet twice, going and returning, and that would be very dangerous. He was also sufficiently self-aware to realize that the quiet of the Annapolis Valley of Nova Scotia, combined with his knowledge of the ongoing war, would unsettle his nerves. He would have no peace of mind despite his peaceful surroundings. He could not shake his thoughts of the front and the sense that he should be there. The war had to be seen to his or its end!

September 8
In the Field

Dearest Sister,

It has been quite a time since I have heard from you or since I have written last so here goes for a few lines. Did you and Ida make out all right at Truro? Have each of you got a school for the coming year? Why don't you exert yourself to get in some place except the back-water ones?

The work I am doing now has quite a degree of importance and while not being without a certain degree of danger, has its good points, being practically left to my own initiative. I wrote a letter to Viola and practically gave her a calling down for being sick. It doesn't seem possible for the snappy eyed cousin of mine to be sick. Last night I got a parcel from M. M. Poole containing 20 packages of cigarettes of the very best quality. I smoke few cigs, but like a pipe and tell dad to send me out a few packages of Dill's Best. I had some photos taken the other day and if any are good I will send one along. The weather has been passing fair the last few days. I hope it will keep so as my work calls me out at any time in connection with mechanical maintenance of an advanced light railway. How is it that Bob and Carl never get sent out to France? They had better never enlisted in my mind, it will surprise some of us at the finish of the war—the number of Canadian heroes there will be!

I felt pretty rotten coming back from leave but soon got used to the routine again. I am now as cheerful as ever, so if I sound like a sepulchre sometimes, why don't think anything of it. Really though, if it were not for the dangers of the Atlantic, why I would put in for three months furlough and, of course I would get it. Anyway, the quiet of the valley would get on my nerves I'm afraid. I am going to give you my address again. Gee, it would be a surprise if I ever got a letter really addressed right. 46277 E. A. Poole Canadian Corps Cyclist Battalion, C Coy BEF—that is quite enough to find me anywhere I may be. I hope this finds you as it leaves me, in good health and spirits.

With loving thoughts to all at home, from your brother E. A. P.

Out of the blue, Eugene's letter of mid-September reflects a considerable upturn in spirits and reveals the reason: he has a girl he writes in England. To mention her to his mother meant that the relationship was a serious one. Combined with this is his interest in photos of his sisters whom he has not seen in over three years and a request, twice stated, to be filled in on all the little personal details of home life. Clearly, Eugene now has a new outlook on matters and a renewed perspective on the possibilities of his life.

 September 15
France

Dear Mother,

It has been some little time since I last heard from anyone home. I haven't been worrying any as I know the mails are not very regular but hope you have been getting along nicely and that my mail reaches you once in a while.

I am in a position now where I have more leisure and inclination to write than I used to have, besides I am a seasoned veteran now and have gradually gotten over my spasmodic ways. There used to be times when I didn't write a letter once a month, but I have improved with age. For the most part, people in Canada get tired of writing to a person who has been away so long, but I correspond with a nice girl in England. Miss Gwendoline Dowd at Ichburgh Iver Heath Bucks. Perhaps one of the girls would like to send a card. If I remember rightly I told you my work in a former letter, but no matter. I am quite well off and wish for nothing better under present circumstances.

Do you receive my assignment regularly now? I sincerely hope that it is of some use to you. I have several hundred dollars in deferred pay owing to me not having made it sooner. The weather has been pretty good lately, better than some time back when I used to get soaked and dry again about three times a day. I had some photos taken the other day. I will send one when they arrive to compare with former ones and while I think of it, please look up the old Bible and let me know what year I was born in, 1890 or 1891? One has so many different ages in the army it's hard to be sure. I wrote to Vera or Ida not long ago. I forgot which. I wish the girls would have some pictures taken. I would like to see how pretty they have all grown in these three years or over. Mother, I never have much news but please make the most of the little personals.

I don't believe I received the last bunch of Monitors you sent, but I remember a Methodist minister writing on the "tot of rum" temperance question etc.,—perfectly sickening and as narrow minded as you would expect from such. Personally, I seldom see it [the rum ration] but the use of it is sanctioned by Medical Authority and is about the only thing to restore circulation after standing in a cold, wet, trench for long. However this is not intended as a lecture so don't be alarmed. Write and tell me all the home doings please. They interest me more than the temperance question or the future history of Europe. What do the people home think of the likelihood of their becoming conscripts? I expect we will have a new thing in Canadian records—the conscientious objector—well we all have our objections! Does father keep fit and well, that's the only thing that ever troubles me. I must go to bed as it is high time.

Love to all at home. E. A. Poole

In late September, mostly in reply to questions he had been asked, Eugene pens a newsy letter to his sister Vera. "Yes," he received her letter and the box of fudge; "no," the papers (personal documents) did not arrive at Dr Olsen's, and does grandmother ever speak of him? Although he does not receive more parcels than his chums, he nonetheless complies with his aunt's request and provides another man's name to whom she could send a parcel. Surely this act of kindness and generosity reflects well on a certain lady's nephew!

September 22
France

Dear Sister,

Number I received safely last night. I am writing a brief letter in reply before going to bed. I am somewhat tired as I have had a very busy and tiring day, but it will make sleep more pleasant I hope. I was glad to hear that you were pleased with the prospects of your school for the ensuing year and that you have a good home to live in. From your description of the place it should be beautiful and that farthermost hill must have very high trees or is it in the highest hill? One thing impressed me about your letter, the address was correct in every detail, though in Ida's the old order was simply changed. I was pleased to get a picture of Ida, she looks better than I would have imagined. The various papers that I had asked for never reached me and I don't believe reached Dr Olsen either. However, I am quite alright without them when the time comes.

Aunt Elna's request rather appealed to my sense of humour as amongst the boys, I know not one gets fewer parcels than I, still I will submit the following name for her approval. Lance Corporal Wallace Millar, Can Corps Cyclist Batt, C Coy CEF. Please remember me to her if you happen to be writing. Does Grandma ever mention my name? I would like to have her think well of me because after all she was always decent to us kids and you remember how we always looked for the paper bag! Well I haven't much to say tonight, but I may have some news in my next letter. I received the box of fudge and it was exceptionally good.

Your loving brother, E A Poole

The Battle of Passchendaele Ridge

By October 1917, British Empire forces, under the overall command of Field Marshal Haig, had been engaged in the battle for Passchendaele ridge for several months. After his British forces had been exhausted and bled dry, Haig sent in the ANZACS—the troops from Australia and New Zealand. They, too, had been slaughtered. Haig finally turned to his last remaining tried and true shock troops—the Canadians—to finish the job. The Canadian Corps commander, General Arthur Currie, did not want his troops to fight at Passchendaele, gauging the objective to be of little permanent value and the potential cost altogether too high. Currie argued against using his crack Canadian troops to finish Haig's quest, especially given the conditions of the battlefield.

By October, millions of shells had destroyed the low-lying area's drainage system, and it had rained for weeks on end. The battlefield was an indescribable wasteland of shell holes, war waste, body parts, and mud. The mud was so deep that men and entire teams of horses sank out of sight. Worse, there was no cover or shelter—trenches and dugouts were impossible to construct or occupy for all was mud and water. The Germans observed all approaches from Passchendaele Ridge and could shell everyone and everything with impunity. General Currie protested, and most likely would have been dismissed had he not been the Canadian Corps commander. Despite Currie's protests, the Canadians had to go. If they had to go, Currie insisted on several weeks' preparation time so as to lessen expected casualties. Currie and his Canadians were granted this brief reprieve by Field Marshal Haig.

To allow movement forward, an entire system of duckboard walkways had to be laid down and constantly repaired—after German shellfire destroyed them. For its part, the Canadian artillery fired in support of the infantry from emplacements clearly visible to the Germans. The Canadian guns had to be placed on timber platforms which lowered with every discharge until they sank beneath the surface. The actual attack involved the Canadian soldiers slogging forward from shell hole to shell hole in knee-deep mud under constant machine-gun and shellfire. Of the hardened veterans who survived, it was common for them to refer to Vimy Ridge as an actual battle, but to their experience at Passchendaele as nothing short of a collective embrace of suicide. Before the battle, General Currie had estimated a cost of sixteen thousand Canadian casualties in order to achieve Haig's objectives. Even with the professionalism, determination, and sacrifice of his Canadian Corps troops, Currie's estimate proved sadly correct.

Eugene writes two letters during the Passchendaele campaign, one on October 27 and another on November 7. He says nothing of the horrors which were transpiring. The only hint is the sudden appearance of the term "Flanders" as his location instead of the more familiar "France." It is indeed the almost complete absence of reference as to where he is, what he is doing, and what the Canadians are up to which is so striking. On October 27, he simply says he has "had scarce time to write lately," and on November 7 that "you can see by the papers the movement of the Canadians." The Battalion War Diary is more revealing. It records that they arrived in the Ypres area near the battle on October 17. From October 29 to 31, German planes dropped bombs on their rear area camp nightly. On November 1, the cyclists suffered five wounded and two gassed; on November 2, one wounded; on November 3, one wounded and one gassed. On November 6, the ridge was taken, but again on November 9, there was one killed and two wounded. The Battalion Diary also records that, by November 8, they had escorted 32 German officers and 745 other ranks as prisoners to the POW cages. It must be remembered that the cyclists were not a front-line infantry battalion attacking the Germans in this battle; they were in a close-support role. What was happening was shocking even by First World War standards. It is little wonder that it left a man from Bridgetown stunned and silenced.

October 27
Flanders

Dear Sister,

I received your letter some time back. I have had scarce time to write lately but will dash off a few lines tonight so that you will know that I am alright. Vera and Ida write quite regularly and it's a real pleasure getting news from them. I was very pleased over your success in gardening etc and that you had a chance to see the public gardens in Halifax. They are not very extensive compared to some in the USA but are beautiful nevertheless. You would do well to take up the study of French thoroughly. It is quite simple and a very useful language. I received a dandy box of fudge from Ida not long ago, it was much appreciated. About my assignment; you should receive $20.00 per month if you do not get that amount let me know or write to Ottawa. If you ever are at a loss what to do with a few dollars, why I keep a pocket for such. Well I must quit as I have some more notes to write.

Your loving brother, E. A. Poole.

Again on November 7, despite the hell he was experiencing, Eugene manages to keep matters light and his sense of humour intact. He will say nothing about the "Canadians' movements" and thus spare the censors the necessity of crossing his words out. All letters were censored by each unit's junior officers, but the greatest censors were the men themselves, who wished to spare their loved ones undue stress and worry. Besides, when all was said and done, most men found Passchendaele an experience beyond words and their powers of description.

November 7
Flanders

Dear Sister [Leila],

Your letters reached me last night, one from Ida as well and just recently from Vera and a parcel from her today so I am doing well in this war. I was very glad to receive you lengthy epistle though I consider them more interesting than anything. I beg your pardon, I read your letter wrong, it was styled interesting after all, my mistake! Really I hadn't noticed that you were being particularly showered with my correspondence. I was afraid that I was getting slow with it. You seem to have given Miss Van Buskirk (was that the name?) a very wrong impression of me. I will enclose a short note telling her the truth. You girls are hopeless in your ideal, if or when, I am it, though I will try and live up to it a little bit. This cigar I am smoking is rather decent and the men are passing remarks about the bad smell, having none to smoke themselves as it has no brother. I was interested to know that Ida has a particular friend. Vera though has had her meeting her fate for some time. It is a different fellow this time. As for the girl I mentioned, she's a decent kid, but merely platonic and do you think that I have a softening of the brain—"Gwenie" indeed! Well I understand that by some strange magic you have grown into a pretty girl. I hope to see for myself some day. You can see by the papers the movement of the Canadians. I never mention anything, then nothing is ever crossed out. The coming winter doesn't appeal to me but I guess I shall stand it. I hope you will like the pictures though they are rotten. Mother wrote a great letter. She must be expecting a good xmas present. It's worth it anyway. I must quit and fix up the note, picture, etc.

Yours lovingly E. A. Poole.

Hints of what had transpired at Passchendaele appear a month later. Having returned to France after their time in Flanders, Eugene speaks of reinforcements, the challenges of training new men, and his attempt to contract the measles.

December 13
France

Dear Sister,

It's about time that I sent you a few lines. I believe you should notice that the heading is different from the last one. Your letter and parcel previous to that arrived safely as did Vera's. Mother's xmas box also arrived on the 12th. It was a marvel of compact neatness and arrived in as good a condition as the day it was packed.

Leila wrote me a very interesting letter filled with home items, it seems funny that she should have the measles again. I snuffed the letter several times in the hopes of catching them myself but have no hopes. Tomorrow I am up for inoculation again as near as I can figure it will be the 9th time. It is a great prevention of disease but I would just as well leave and be excused. We have been having a very quiet time lately getting our battalion reinforced etc and filling in the rest with almost constant training, necessary but a considerable bore.

I had a talk with Harry Starrett or Lt Starrett as I shall say. He is in charge of a platoon in B Coy, he is the same Harry. I expect it's up to me to congratulate you if you're engaged to your Bryson. Knowing you to be the girl you are, it's all right of course, but perfectly silly to an old bachelor like myself. On xmas day we are having a "bonne Fete" a regular old feed, I believe. I was pleased to hear that Henry got a moose, I would like a good piece of it in front of me at the present time. My xmas presents were not many this year as I have spent my money being around towns this year. I wish I could get permission to go to Canada if only to skim around the lake with you this winter on skates. I have forgotten the art by this time. Well, I must close before you can decode this as I have written it by firelight.

Your loving brother, E. A. Poole

The new men Eugene mentions were, of course, replacements for those killed and wounded at Passchendaele. By this stage of the war, due to the increasingly technical nature of signalling and linesman duties, additional on-site training was required. New men also required a period to acclimatize to actual front-line conditions before they were of much practical use. He comments on this, as well as on his dwindling number of chums in his December 22 letter to his mother. He also comments on family matters, such as Ida's boyfriend, Uncle Olsen's trip, and his hoped for leave to Paris. Finally, he apologizes to his mother for not having the funds to buy much in the way of Christmas gifts this year.

December 22
France

Dear Mother,

Your letters and parcels were received in good time and everything in perfect condition. I have been having a very good time for the past three weeks and expect to have a jolly xmas as all arrangements have been made for a big day. Owing to being back from the line so long this year I have selfishly spent my money so I have not been able to send many xmas souvenirs but I hope you will forgive me. Last year I spent xmas in a dug-out, quite a change this year. I have received a lot of mail lately from home and also a nice letter from grandma. I answered Mrs Laytes parcel with a note. The weather has been very cold and frosty here for some time but it's much better than rain, though hard to get one's head out of the blankets mornings. Almost all of our coy [company] are strangers to me now, the old boys fade away in various ways, there are only about five of us left in my platoon. When you speak of leave to Canada did you ever enquire if you could make application yourself through Canada, perhaps you could think of some excuse. In about a month I expect to go to Paris for two weeks. My available credit is not very large, if it would be possible for you to send me some it would help and I could make it up later by remittance. Leila wrote a nice letter, of course, it didn't upset me much, perhaps she was serious, I am sure she was innocent. Ida must have a very nice boy, I am certain he would have to be or she would not like him. Of course I am skeptical as ever, but I am not quite hopeless, though Uncle Olsen says I am incorrigible! He had a very pleasant time in the States and reached England safely. Well, I must close now as I have a few letters to write.

Your loving son, E. A. Poole

1918

At the very end of 1917, the dreaded, but almost statistically inevitable, happened: Eugene's father received a Western Union telegram. Something significant had happened to Eugene; was he dead? missing? wounded? All these years later, we can only imagine the worry and anxiety with which the telegram was received and opened.

> J F Poole, Bridgetown N.S. Sincerely regret to inform you 46277 Pte Eugene A Poole officially reported admitted eleventh Field Ambulance. December twenty ninth 1917 Gunshot wound right thigh.

Relief, indeed: only a gunshot wound to the thigh. Amazingly, the Battalion War Diary, which does not often mention specific minor injuries, records this incident. As it turned out, the cyclists were being employed a great deal at this point as night-time wiring parties. A few officers and several dozen men would go out into no man's land in the dark to erect elaborate mazes of barbed wire in front of their own trenches. The Diary records that, on December 28, "both parties on the same wiring work as before, one man in wiring party wounded in thigh by a machine gun bullet." But did the telegram tell Eugene's family the full story? Was this an accurate report? As things turned out, it was. Eugene wrote his mother from hospital as soon as he could.

January 5

Dearest Mother,

You will have received official notice by this time that I have been wounded, but don't let it worry you any as it is very slight. Just a clean machine gun bullet which "winged" my thigh—nearly missed me as a matter of fact. It means a few weeks rest down the line this time [within the Canadian hospital system in France], that is all I can hope for, though England would look good for the winter. It was only my second night up the line after a month's rest so I am very lucky indeed. I had just written to you that morning so if the postman collected it off my bed you will get it ahead of this. This is a very personal letter—all about myself, but I merely wanted you to know that I am OK and well looked after at the hospital. Another old timer has the cot beside mine—a 2nd Canadian Infantry Battalion man and we have a good time.

Love to all from your son, and only, E. A. Poole.

Amazingly, we have a record of Eugene's account of this incident. While on leave in September 1918, Eugene related to his uncle, Dr Olsen, the details of his wounding and recovery.

> Eugene, along with a number of other cyclists, was carrying some irons for the purpose of putting up barbed wire obstructions in front of the enemy. When all of a sudden he felt as though someone had struck him from behind and he dropped to a sitting position. He whispered to the man behind him, "what are you doing?" But the other soldier, who had heard the whiz of the machine gun bullet, at once cut open his trouser and tried to stop the hemorrhage, which fortunately was not too great. With the aid of a chum, he walked about half a mile to the outpost station of the field ambulance where he received first aid treatment. After this he was carried on a stretcher to the Casualty Clearing Station, where he arrived in a little more than half an hour after he was shot. The bullet only grazed the upper end of the femur, but nevertheless caused a wound that took three months to heal. The first thing that was done to him at the Casualty Clearing Station was the administration of anti-tetanic serum in his left

arm. Up to that time he had felt no great pain for the wound had stunned him. Eugene says he had much more pain from the injection in the arm than he ever had from the bullet wound. The arm swelled up and was very painful for two days, but undoubtedly saved him from coming down with tetanus. Nevertheless there must have been some kind of poison for there was a black band on the outside of his thigh reaching up to his armpit and fully four inches in breadth. In spite of all this he made a good recovery

Being hospitalized not surprisingly generated a lot of letters to Eugene during his recuperation. Writing to two of his sisters a month later, he speaks of having received letters from grandma, his Uncle Olsen in England, and "all three of my sisters." All these letters and lying in the hospital also meant Eugene had time to write back. While approving of what Ida tells him of her fiancé, he offers some advice to them both. It would be best if her man tempered his career ambitions and avoided that "other" service—namely, the air force—and his chances of coming home to her will be better! Overall, his tone is now considerably more relaxed than before. He even employs a new nickname for himself: Chips.

February 4
France

Dearest Sister Ida,

Your letter was rather slow in reaching me owing to several shifts that I have made. I was very glad to receive it and to know that you had a flying visit home. My mail all reached me in a shower and letters from all three of my sisters. Your description of your fiance quite satisfies me, I can quite believe he is a clever and sensible young man. Only Ida, the next time you write to him tell him not to let his ambition carry him too far in the branch you previously mentioned. There is plenty of scope in his own line and a better opportunity of him coming back to you. I was grieved to hear of George Banks being killed. It's rough on his father for the old man cared a lot about him for all his sternness.

I expect you have had all kinds of skating etc., this winter with the lakes right at your door. For the last month I have been enjoying summer weather. We have been playing baseball here at this camp. Personally, I haven't played much till lately, but am all right for the old game now, but believe me I would enjoy having on my old skates again. This is the fourth winter that I have been away from the ice.

Wynn [his English girl] wrote and told me that she had received a letter from you. She was very pleased about it too. She is a clerk in the APC and an indispensible one too as she has recently been singled out for special work. Dr Olsen wrote me telling me to be sure and spend my next leave with him. He was very sorry to know that I had received such a major wound after me telling him that the bullet almost missed me. I must write Leila a few lines, I have written to Vera quite recently as I will wait a few days.

"Au Revoir" from you loving brother, Chips

Writing to his younger sister Leila the same day, Eugene teases her as he comments on a photo she has sent. He was looking for pigtails, but she is now four years older than when he last saw her. Not only has he missed four winters of skating on the lakes of Nova Scotia, but also four years of family life, including the maturing of his young sister. Eugene's war has indeed dragged on for a long while.

February 4
France

Dear Baby Sister,

I have just written a short letter to Ida and will now try and scribble a few lines to you. Your photo was the most amazing thing. I looked at it a long while and thought that it must be someone I knew, or need to know, it took some figuring to realize that you were in your eighteenth year. I was looking for a pigtail at least! All of my letters simply cried of snow and ice, and here I am enjoying weather almost like summer, however I could enjoy a little of that same ice and snow.

Grandma wrote me a nice letter and I have since answered it, but I never answered Viola's last one, beautiful as it was. I would like to write to all of my merry cousins though, when you see them tell them that. I think of them very often. I was planning to go on leave to Paris just before I got hit but I will give up the idea now and go to blighty instead. Paris is a wonderful city but a bit gay for an old batch like me, and I have some pretty nice friends in England. Also uncle A. B. Olsen and aunt Mary but (M. Poole Olsen M.D. F.R.C.S.) is still in America. It's hard to realize that they hold all kinds of degrees to see them in private life.

I am sorry that you didn't see Miss Van Buskirk. I am sure that I should have had a good laugh over your recording of the incident. Mother thought that I would take you quite seriously in your discourse about her. Leila, I am not laughing at you, but what a game—everyone splitting on the other person.

Well so long for this time, with love and to all, Your Brother Chips.

Over a month later, Eugene pens a quick note to his sister Ida. He is better now. He has to return to base camp and then to his battalion, but he has leave coming to him and so his spirits are high. He also admits that he regrets having to leave his convalescent environment—it has been a good place and a great break as well as a rest. The Empire's hospital services had improved a great deal by early 1918. Advances had been made in healing both bodies and minds. Sadly, before the war's end, there would be many more patients on which to hone their skills.

March 16
France

Dearest sister Ida,

I have just scribbled a few lines to Vera and I will send you a note also, as I am leaving for the base tomorrow where I shall soon be sent to my battalion. It will not be long now before I shall be going on leave. From all I can hear and read one is pretty nearly as safe in this country provided one is not too near the line of course. This letter is being written while there is a service going on (in the Soldiers' Christian Association, like the YMCA) so if I write down some of the Perthshire experience of the speaker, pardon me. Wynn was so pleased with your letter that she sent it on for me to read. It was pretty decent of you to write to her. Have you gotten any word when Selden sails for France? If I knew his address, I might look him up when I go on leave. My uncle Olsen wants me to spend my leave with him and Wynn's mother tells me to make right for Uxbridge—maybe I shall split the difference successfully. I will enclose one of these snaps or photos which like most French pictures are as musty as the studio they take them in. So long for this time, I will write later. It makes me rather homesick leaving here; it's a bon place.

Your loving brother, E. A. Poole

Sadly, Eugene's hoped-for leave was not to be. On March 21, 1918, the Germans launched a massive attack on the British army in France. This was the first of several offensives designed to destroy the Allied armies, or at least break their will to continue and to render their positions militarily untenable so that they would sue for peace. As the Empire's forces reeled backwards under the assault, all leave was cancelled. Eugene returned to his unit just a few days after the offensive began. Given the situation, Eugene's spirits are not too low; as a First Contingent man, however, he is thinking out loud about legitimate means to escape any further time at the front.

March 31
France

Dearest sister Leila,

Just arrived back to the battalion two days ago with the cheerful prospect in front of me, chiefly—all leave stopped. I should have been away a month ago if I had been here. Do you suppose Hazel Van Buskirk would marry me if I asked her nicely? It's about the only way I can think of to get to Canada on leave. The few married men of the First Contingent have gone back. I wish I had been in bondage at the time. It was great down in the south of France where I was. I should like to have spent my time there for the rest of the war, but unfortunately they have a policy of making you fit around that part of the country sur-mer. The pictures of your girls were fine and I was very pleased to get them. It is raining out again or yet, I should say, though it is cheerful enough in here [the YMCA hut] with the band playing. What would you like when I go on leave in lieu of no present at xmas time? I hope everything is OK at home. Tell father to put in application for me to come home and help him as I should be able to get it—lots of the old boys are getting back. He must need my help anyway. This note does not sound very cheerful but I feel pretty good at that and might be a lot worse off.

Yours with love to all at home, E. A. Poole.

Eugene's hope for leave back to Canada was a reasonable one for a First Contingent man. He was unable to know the bigger picture, however, and thus was unaware of the severity of the situation. The Germans had advanced significantly, and whether or not they could be stopped in time remained an open question. He pens a note to Vera a few days later, talking about socks, the difficulty of adjusting to being back at it, and the fact that his chum did receive the parcel from aunt Alma! "Jack Canuck" is Eugene's version of "Johnny Canuck," a personification of the nation.

April 4
France

Dear Sister,

When I come to think of it I have rather neglected writing to you lately. I try to write to some of you about once a week or fortnight at least. Ida sent me a dandy pair of socks. I am getting stocked up a bit now in that line. We quite often receive a pair from the Red Cross Society and they are the only kind I can wear with comfort. While you have been having a very severe winter, the season here has been unusual in warmth and sunshine with hardly enough cold days to let us know it's winter. I have been back a few days now and find it a bit different than playing ball or else doing nothing at a convalescent camp. I must try and see if I can get a special leave to Canada but I don't have much idea of getting it. Also I must ask "Jack Canuck" how some of the fellows around home manage to stick it so long after joining up at all? "Pack" Anderson is back now or rather DeBlois Anderson, Capt. DSO is, I believe. You have met him or his sister Nora at least. He is a great lad. I have met him out here quite a lot and I also met his cousin after Passchendaele. He wished to be remembered to all at home. I must quit now and straighten up my bed. I am writing this lying on my back in bed. Wallace Miller received a parcel from aunt Alma all right, he told me. He wished me to thank her again for him though he acknowledged it at the time.

Your loving brother, E. A. Poole

The German offensive continued to rage into April and Eugene pens a quick note to his sister Vera. He tells her of cancelled leave, confusion and in the midst of it all answers a query about what should go in a care package from an uncle in the USA. Surely an amazing diversity of matters to cover given the circumstances.

April 13
France

Dear Vera,

Your letter and parcel arrived a few days ago. Everything was in good condition and I enjoyed it very much. I have forgotten uncle Mayor's address. That is why I have not written to him. He is very good and I cannot thank him enough for his kindness. What I would like from him most I don't know. You might tell him discreetly that my pay in dollars is about 8 a month and the YMCA charges anything. Too much is wasted in postage etc in a parcel from the States. Still they are nice things to get for all that. You will be surprised to hear that I was prevented from going on leave as all U.K. leave was cancelled. Too much is doing here at present for any such luxuries (as leave) and I don't have any idea when it will open up again. Fritz is putting up a strong offensive and will take some stopping, but everything should come all right soon, I hope. Well everything is in confusion and noisy here tonight so will close.

Just wanted to let you know I am alright. E. A. Poole

The German offensive of spring 1918 was the most serious threat the Allies had faced. By May, despite significant German gains and heavy losses on both sides, the exhausted armies reached another stalemate. After almost two months of silence, Eugene writes his sister again. He admits to an absence of motivation with respect to writing, a sin of omission which has gotten him into hot water with his English girlfriend. His reference to the inequalities of leave were true and a running sore point between the officers and all other ranks. Eugene's phrase, "owing to a slight misfortune," causing three men to go twenty-eight months without leave, most likely refers to a disciplinary infraction. Such an offence was, in the overall scheme of things, minor, but nonetheless sufficient from the army's perspective to deny the men their regular leave rotation.

June 11
France

Dear Sister,

It has been a long while since I have written, so I must try and send off a few lines. I have been having a pretty soft time lately, plenty of parades etc but no particular element of danger. The old French villages are pretty good places to live in though troops constantly billeted in them for several years spoil it some. I have never written to Sheldon. I have been expecting to see him most any time, but I shall meet him before long. I will wait til he has a chance to acclimatize a bit. Leave is a very slow affair at present. I am not worrying about it at all. We have three men who, owing to a slight misfortune, have been twenty-eight months without leave. Still, one of our officers who has been out five months, went on regular leave the other day.

In the last letter I got from Wynn she was pretty sore at the way I postponed writing but it can't be done if the spirit won't move. I feel in good health and spirits but what is there to spiel about that I haven't said before? Of course it's pretty selfish as I like to hear from home. The weather keeps perfect though the roads are very dusty. Next time you write to Seldon ask him what he thinks of Fritz's rubber gun. Well excuse the brevity and nothingness of this note.

Your loving brother, Eugene

Eugene forces himself to catch up on his letter writing, and pens one to another sister the next day. One hopes his comments on her knitting prowess were taken humorously. As for his sore leg from playing sports, the army was hardening the troops for a big push upcoming in August. Sports were a great means of increasing physical fitness without the men endlessly grumbling about PT (physical training) and route marches.

June 12
France

Dear Sister,

My letters are few and far between these days but my supply of news is very small also. We have been having it very soft for some time and I am feeling in fine form except that I have a stiff leg from running in the battalion sports. The weather has been fine for a long time—only the dust on the road is annoying.

I expect by the time you receive this you will be about ready to start home on summer holidays. It is possible that I may get a holiday myself this summer but I am not banking on it very strong. The socks you sent were O.K. Please thank Mrs Wall for me for the part she played in their construction—I can hardly imagine you as a successful knitter, as it must be a bit tedious. I expect to see Seldon some of these days but at present the IInd F.A. [Field Artillery] is some distance from here. Mrs Burke sent me a decent letter a while back which I have never answered yet. If you happen to be writing please apologize for me will you?

Well so long and try and have a good time this summer, as ever, E. A. Poole

Shortly after writing his sisters, Eugene had an outbreak of severe impetigo which landed him in hospital. Such skin diseases were common among the troops, for living conditions at the front were anything but sanitary. He thanks his three sisters profusely for their letters and the cheerfulness and vitality of their goings on. He is recovering well, and worries about matters at home: did his father take a break from work to go fishing? He also teases his sister about the opportunity of wearing pants and doing what was considered "men's work." He has seen many instances of this in England, and then recalls that she had apparently passed on just such an opportunity the previous summer.

June 26
France

Dear Sister,

I have just read your combined letters, yours and Leila's and was pleased with the joyous way she has of living. It is a great thing to be able to enjoy each little experience with all the innocence of youth. You and Vera are the same too though your duties must be very exacting. With the common sense you all have it makes a pleasant combination. It is too bad that you have never had the opportunity of taking up music to the extent you wish, try and console yourself with the fact that you are really as good as you are. How much would a year at the seminary cost you? Aunt Bert and Lulu wrote to me. It was a pleasant surprise though there was a difference of eleven days in the two letters enclosed. Lulu informs me that she is sixteen, 5ft, 3 inches and 120 lbs. She also asks about my possible sweethearts in foreign lands, so I think she must be growing up all right. I have also written to Bryson. I would have done so before but expected to go up and see him but I have been in the hospital for a couple of weeks. I had a nice little outbreak which unfortunately is quite well now. I shouldn't say that but I have no love for the training we have in our rest periods, and this has been a change.

I expect you will be about ready for vacation by the time you get this. It is possible I may get leave by August, though I never let a small matter like that worry me. Your letters are all so cheerful from home these days it's a pleasure to get them. I am feeling fine these days too though I lack the expression somehow. I do hope father went down for a fishing trip. His pleasures can't be any too many with all he does. The party they had out to the lakes must have been some trip for the girls.

Wait till the girls wear pants in Canada like they do in England though. What occupation do you propose putting in for under the new man / women power in Canada? It is no joke in England at present and it may be a serious question in Canada soon, so watch out for your opportunity. I forgot your last summer vacation though, pardon me. I forgot that opportunity had not found you in the back yard.

Please forgive the craziness of this, from your loving brother, Eugene.

On August 8, 1918, it was time for the Allies to push back. The over-extended and weakened German forces were a tempting target, but no pushover. All along the Western Front, the Allied armies attacked. The Canadian Corps was secretly transferred to the Amiens front in France and attacked with great success on the opening day of the offensive and the days following. The Canadian advance was measured in miles instead of the usual metres, but the cost of such success was high: the Canadian Corps would suffer 30 percent of all its Great War casualties over the next one hundred days. The success in early August was followed by more pitched battles at month's end and into early September. Thankfully, Eugene was on leave at the end of August and escaped the dangers of the Battle of Arras and the breaking of the Drocourt-Quéant Line on September 2. At the end of his leave, Eugene briefly visited his uncle, Dr Olsen. The dear doctor had the presence of mind to record Eugene's account of the breakthrough Battle of Amiens (August 8–14), which he had experienced.

> The particular duty of the cyclist corps in this push was to go forward in small groups to various villages and clear them of any Germans that might have been left behind. This meant that the cyclists were in advance of the infantry anywhere from a mile to a mile and a half.
>
> Just before going in to battle the men had a good feed. Then they were ordered to take all the food that they could possibly

carry in their haversacks. These supplies sufficed them for two days. Although on the second day they were just a little short of food and felt a little pinched in that regard. The food Eugene took in his pack was several tins of baked beans, a lot of baked potatoes in their jackets, a small bottle of pickles, heaps of bread and butter and a tin of Californian pears which he bought at the Y.M.C.A. for one and a half francs. He thought it held about two pints. Bully beef was offered to him in abundance but he does not care for it at all.

Eugene says the battle of Amiens was the experience of his life. He never saw so many Germans before and he says it was most amusing at times to see them on the run. He says he winged several with his own rifle. At any rate, he saw them drop so something must have happened. The enemy were so taken by surprise that they did not have much time to do much shelling. They barely heard the enemy shells and their big guns appeared to have been silent, at least in that sector of the line where Eugene was working. In their wild flight the enemy left behind stores of all kinds—guns (small and large) and trinkets of one sort and another. Among the souvenirs and trinkets Eugene picked up on the battlefield was a splendid and perfect prismatic binocular with compass, worth, at the very least 15 or 20, but as he had no use for it he sold it for 150 francs. He also got an old fashioned German pipe with a long fancy stem and dangling tassels, which he said weighed half a pound or more that he sold for 10 francs. He also picked up a full blooded German dachshund which he captured in a German dugout It was a perfect beauty with glistening black fur like that of a seal and was evidently a valuable animal. The dog wore a collar with a name, Eugene explained, at least a yard long that he did not attempt to spell or pronounce. To the collar was attached a light, strong, steel chain. As his cyclist battalion had no mascot or pet, he presented this dog to them, so that he will see it again when he returns to his battalion this week. Eugene is very fond of the dog and proud of its capture.

He picked up many other trinkets including a German steel helmet but as it weighed a great deal he did not carry it far.

On the first night after the start of the attack there was a brief halt so Eugene and the rest got a little sleep, but it was both fitful and restless on account of the great excitement. The next day the experience was very much like that of the first day, rushing forward in small groups to clean the villages of the final remnant of the enemy, one after another. Again the enemy was rushing forward wildly and there was scarcely any rear-guard action, and no heavy guns of the Germans were in action. They captured a lot of guns and their ammunition, sometimes with a shell in the gun all ready to be fired. Eugene tells me that most of the guns captured, as far as he could observe, were in perfect condition.

The second night after starting the push, Eugene found himself at a very dangerous outpost in company with the rest of his party. But, fortunately, the unhealthiness of the post was not discovered until the danger was past. They got no sleep that night for they were kept busy attending to the duties of various sorts. A German officer strode into the place in a perfectly innocent fashion, never dreaming that it was occupied by the Canadians and it was a simple matter to capture him. Again, some German soldiers, also quite innocent as to the change in the control of this particular outpost, were seen wheeling barrows, probably full of ammunition. They, of course, thought that the place was still in the hands of the Germans but they soon found themselves under the protection of the Canadians. This is an indication of both the speed and continuing development of the advance.

This was the first time that Eugene and his corps went into action on their bicycles. They had good use of them too and were thus enabled to make rapid progress which they otherwise could not have done. When he was in the Vimy Ridge attach in the spring of 1917, the bicycles were left behind and the corps was put on machine guns and of course advanced on foot.

After the rush of the first few days was over there was a general clean up of both body and clothing, polishing of buttons and boots, shaving etc so as to be ready for inspection. His battalion numbered approximately 275 men and out of this number only two were killed and thirty wounded during the first three days of the push. He thinks that this exceedingly small loss was a very fair average for the other battalions as far as he could hear. They lost no prisoners and although his cycling battalion was not supposed to take any prisoners they were simply obliged to gather up a few which came their way. The rush of the battle was over by the end of the fourth day and from then on to the 15th, when he was to have leave, he had a relatively quiet time.

In early September, his leave over, Eugene writes his sister. He speaks of snaps, socks, and the advance, but this time he has really big personal news to tell: a ring has been purchased!

September 4
France

Dear Sister,

I have just returned from leave and must tell you first of all that I was too busy and the time too short for me to go down to Hastings much as I would have liked to have gone. All my time that I could get was devoted to the dental chair and I am very glad that I took the opportunity though the expense was considerable. I also bought a ring, which will put the wind up mother as Wynne and I became engaged. You won't need any slush from me to know that she is a very nice kid. I hope she won't regret it, as for me, I'm about half fit for her. Ask uncle what he thinks of her, his opinion should be worth something. I shall ask Shelden to meet her. I think especially if he gets to her home in Uxbridge it would be interesting; Uxbridge by the way is a very likely spot for him to be sent. I expect to join the battalion up the line in the morning. This is a real struggle and the casualties are naturally not few. I will have the strength to face danger fearlessly, I know, because of you girls at home who I am sure are always praying for my safety. Your letter was waiting for me when I got back and I think I appreciated it more than anything I have ever had from home. The socks were on time too and thanks for the gum. I sent the snaps by this same mail on to Winnie who will be pleased to see them and send them back to me later. I hardly understand you letter re Vera Longley [a cousin]. You first say that she is going to teach near you, then that she is going to the Seminary at the opening. I hope I don't appear dense. I must close with my love. I will write home soon and tell mother the situation; her letters are really the most unaffected that I have ever read. I do enjoy one of her rare ones.

Yours as ever, Chip

Engaged! News of such magnitude at a time of such danger necessitated a letter to his mother. Eugene soon penned it.

September 15
France

Dear Mother,

Since last writing home I have been on two weeks leave to England. It was a beautiful season of the year and I enjoyed myself very much in a very proper way. I spent a few days at Caterham and uncle took a day off and we went for an excursion up the river Thames. The rest of my time I put in at the girl's home at Uxbridge. I thought you, being my loving and long suffering mother, might be interested to know that I became engaged while in blighty. The girl is Miss Wynne Dowd or strictly speaking Gwendolyn Margaret Drake Dowd. I don't claim that she's the only girl in the world but I have known her nearly four years and she is a sincere, straight, lovable girl so the only thing you can do is to swallow your lump and give us your blessing. I'm sure she would appreciate a note from you or father. I was pleased to hear from Vera yesterday and to know that she and Ida are so near this year. They are great girls with plenty of ambition. I was very sorry that I could not go down to Hastings to see Shelden. It would have pleased Ida, but my time was more than taken up.

We are having it quiet just now and I escaped a warm time being on leave when I was. We had quite a few casualties but we had some great sport on the Somme with slight loss [August 8]. Try and not worry about me. I feel that I will come through all right. The war will be over in less than two years. Hope everything is OK at home, the snaps were very good. Send a bar of maple sugar and a lb of sugar for porridge in the mornings if you can without too much trouble. It is comical going on leave with a ration book of coupons.

Love to all. Eugene

By Eugene's next letter, in late October, the pace of the war had changed drastically. After the smashing of the German defences along the Canal du Nord in late September, true open warfare had returned. The expanses of no man's land and intricate trench systems were left behind. The Canadian Corps now chased the retreating Germans as hard as they could. Canadian commanders sent their fastest troops, the cyclists, forward in hot and dangerous pursuit. Back in May the entire battalion of cyclists had been trained as two-man Lewis (light) machine-gun teams. During the 100 Days Campaign, the cyclists often worked in tandem with the Canadian Motor Machine Gun Brigade. This unique formation, commanded by General Raymond Bruti-

nel, consisted of his armoured cars brimming with machine guns, the cyclists' Lewis gun teams, and mobile trench mortar teams. The goal was to have a highly mobile unit of intense firepower available to move where it was needed, to support the infantry's attack, and to advance more quickly than previously possible in order to exploit success.

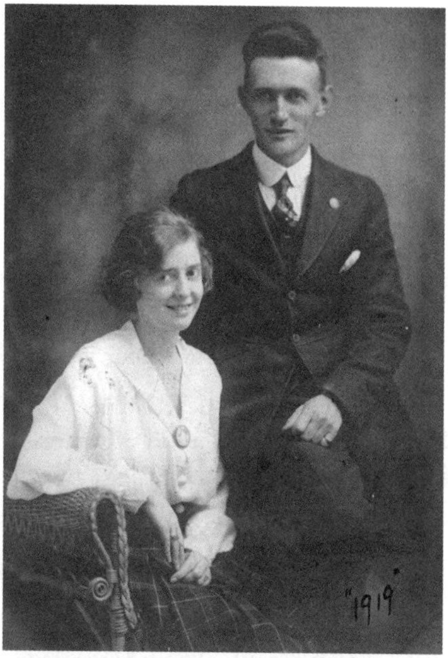

Eugene and Winnie at the time of their marriage. Notice how gaunt Eugene's face is compared to earlier photos—years of active service have taken a toll.

Despite the Allied advances, the German army itself had not been defeated as a viable fighting force. As it retreated in order, however, villages and entire cities that had endured years of occupation were liberated. Eugene writes his eldest sister Vera, telling her about the liberated towns and villages and the excited, recently freed civilians who did not hesitate to show their appreciation and their joy.

October 26

Dear Sister Vera,

I just received your letter dated 13th September. It was quite a while reaching me. You girls write lovely letters. I think the secret must lie in them being so natural. Was your quotation from "Paradise Lost"? It sounded dimly familiar. Armstrong of my unit received your letter all right and started to answer it but while he was away from his pad someone copped the whole thing and left him like most of the rest of us who were without anything to write on. He is on leave at present. His people live in London, so it's going home for him.

The recent advances have been wonderful. It's a joyous sight to see the civilians flocking out to greet our troops when they enter the liberated towns, they have had over four years of bondage and a khaki uniform is a great sight to them—they greet you with a kiss on either cheek. Some of the towns are intact but others are a mass of blown up ruins—Fritz will have a big bill to answer. At present I am not with the battalion but am on the brigade HQ. The house we are living in is not only comfortable but it is luxurious—everything that a person could wish for is there. There are also few civilians in this town. Not long ago I received a letter from Inez Rice, Mrs Austin's sister, Smith Cove. It was a big surprise as I had nearly forgotten her but it was a pleasant surprise and I was quite prompt in answering it for a wonder. I am glad that you and Ida are so near home this year but it's luck that you can appreciate the beauties of nature so well living so far from civilization as you do. I wish sometimes that you would use your wonderful descriptive powers on something that interests you in the nature line to the extent of not over one hundred words. I would send it to the Daily Mail as they have a space every day just for that and I think you would easily compete.

Wyn writes me quite regularly and is feeling fit though working hard at the office only greatly worried over her brother Percy who is in the Australian Infantry.[14] They have not heard from the kid for six weeks or so and he usually writes regularly. Of course, the mail service is handicapped just now [due to the pace of the advance] but not to that extent.

14 It would appear that Wynn's brother had emigrated "Down Under" before the war and had joined the Australian infantry. He apparently survived the war, as the Commonwealth War Graves Commission has no listing of his death.

She was out to see uncle Olsen last Sunday—he is a lovely man. I wish I could meet him just now. He is in Scotland for two weeks.

Ida's fudge arrived and was greatly appreciated by all who were handy. I see by the papers that your supply of sugar is cut down. It's amusing in Blighty, you have a coupon for practically everything. By the time you have visited all the restaurants you feel like going home to a meal. Out at Wyn's place though we had everything one would wish for—it's different if you have place enough to call a farm. Tell Leila to go into French a little seriously and not to think of missing it. I must close this up. Tell Ida I will write before long.

Your loving brother, Eugene

This was Eugene's last letter home before the war ended. While he no doubt wrote his fiancée Wynn in England expressing his thoughts and emotions at the Armistice on November 11, this correspondence has not survived. The end of warfare, however, did not mean the end of life in the army. Eugene was among thousands of Canadian troops who marched into Germany and formed part of an Allied army of occupation in the fall and winter of 1918–19. Eugene's Cyclist Battalion entered Germany on December 9, 1918, and left by train on February 4, 1919. The rationale behind this occupation was to ensure that Germany's new government would capitulate fully to the Allies' harsh treaty terms. Eugene returned to England on March 7, 1919. He was apparently tired of army rules, for upon his return to England and Wynn, he went Absent Without Leave from March 14 to March 22. Although the war was over, the army could not simply overlook such behaviour. He could have been jailed for such action, but his punishment was forfeiture of his "Good Conduct Badge," awarded the previous May, and the loss of fifteen days' pay—a serious financial punishment. Not surprisingly, Eugene mentions none of this in his letters home, two of which survive from 1919; instead they are full of news, future plans, and joyous revelations.

April 4, 1919
Ripon Camp, England
Dear Mother and family,

It has been a long time since I have written home but here it goes for a few lines tonight to let you know that everything is O.K. though the monotony of these rest camps is not pleasant. I am in the north of England and its very beautiful here with many famous places of interest. So many troops though take the joy out of the place—most of them are men of the Rainbow Division that is, they "came after the storm." You will remember the Borums. I met young B on several occasions. He is a very interesting boy, clean minded and a real man. The war has been a wonderful experience to him as he was taken prisoner at the second battle of Ypres [April 1915] so he has had his share of "camp life."

I am disappointed in not being able to sail on the 12th of this month but there are a lot of papers to fix up yet owing to me getting married while on my leave after arriving from France last month. I never thought I should marry but it's done now and I shall do my best in the future. We were married at noon on the 22nd of March and I left for the north on the 4 o'clock train—simply married by courtesy that's all.

Dr Olsen is sailing for America about May. He may look you up. If he does come, look after him to the best of your ability and see that he gets plenty of plain good food but only in the vegetarian line because he has used me mighty decent the times I have been with him.

I expect it will be the middle of summer before I get over. You had better send me a T. Eaton's and Simpson's catalogue so that I can send my order and have my clothes waiting for me. Also [mother,] you will not receive an assignment [of his pay] much longer as I had to transfer it to my wife in order to receive the separation allowance.

Well I must quit now and write another short note, Love to all, Eugene.

May 2, 1919
Seaford Camp, England

Dear Mother,

No doubt you have been expecting me home by this time but it will be another month or two before that happens. I am looking forward to seeing you all again as perhaps you are me, though you will soon get tired of me, I think.

It is very monotonous living around camps here in England or anywhere for that matter though I can't complain too much as I have been on two fifteen days leave since I arrived home from France on March 7th. Wynn and I spent a two weeks honeymoon trip to Shanklin on the Isle of Wight, it's a lovely place and we had a good time though the water was still a bit cool for bathing. You will please be as nice as you can be to Wynn mother. She is a dear girl, really far too good for me. She has never wanted for anything as her mother is quite comfortably off. She is not a spoilt child by any means and is really sensible except that she chose to marry me. I haven't seen the doctor [Uncle Olsen] lately. He may have sailed for America, he was planning to look you up. If you write to me again send it to Wynn's home address as one never is lucky enough to see his mail here at camp. The address is; Ichburgh Farm, Iver Heath, Bucks, Love to all Eugene.

Eugene and Wynn arrived in Canada in August 1919. Family tradition suggests that Wynn received a warm welcome and adjusted well to what had to have been a significant social and cultural shift. Eugene and Wynn lived in the same community as Eugene's parents, Paradise, Nova

Scotia. They had three healthy children: Iris, Barbara, and Gwendolyn. Sadly, by the 1930s, most likely as a result of his war service, especially exposure to gas, Eugene suffered from ill health. He died at the early age of forty-seven on July 8, 1937. His death certificate lists the cause of death as pulmonary tuberculosis. Wynn lived until July 2, 1955.

NURSING SISTER

Pauline D. Balloch

OF CENTREVILLE, NEW BRUNSWICK

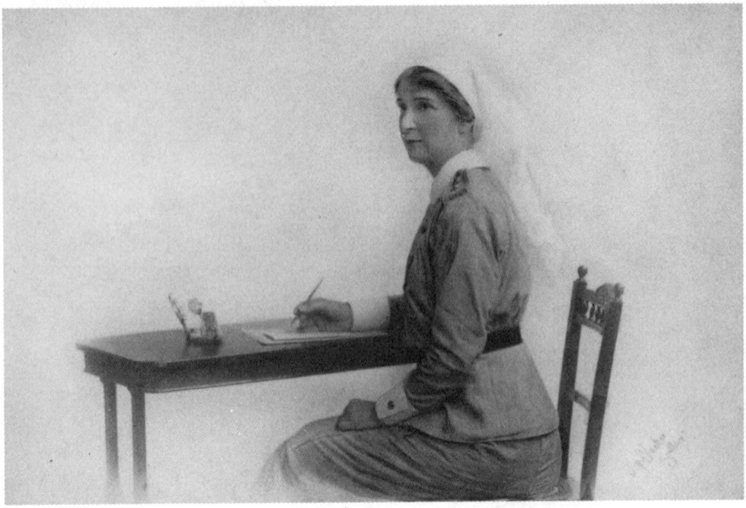

Pauline seated at her desk.

Pauline D. Balloch did not have to go to war. As a thirty-five-year-old nurse, she represented something new in early twentieth century Canada: an educated, single, and financially independent woman. She did not have to be married in order to have either financial security or status. Indeed, marriage, if she desired it, would only have tied her down. As matters stood, she was free to make up her own mind, and she did. In the late spring of 1917, after both Vimy Ridge and the American declaration of war, Pauline joined the Canadian Army Medical Corps. After returning to Canada from work in New York and doing palliative care work with a Mr Bridges in Toronto, Pauline joined up officially on May 2, 1917.

Pauline had significant connections in New Brunswick. Her elderly parents, Robert and Alice Balloch, weighed on her mind. All her surviving letters are addressed to them in Centreville, Carleton County. The first letter appears to postdate Pauline's breaking the news to her parents of her intention to join the CAMC. She speaks of poor old dying Mr Bridges, her purchase of a new outfit for $40, attending a live play with friends in Toronto, *and parish life at the Anglican minister's house in Centreville. Her note ends with comments about the Canadian victory at Arras (Vimy Ridge).*

April 11, 1917

Dearest Dears,

My last letter has been worrying me lest it disturbed you. Truly it would have been better had I not written at all, rather than write at such a time. Caring for poor old Mr Bridges had just about robbed me of all sense of proportion; the first week was extremely hard—he gave me no rest day or night and there was no retreat; irrational, headstrong, heavy, though small, but on Saturday night relief came and since I have been doing only day duty. He cannot get better but may linger sometime. As a case I cannot call him interesting. His daughter is very nice.

My spring suit is lovely. It cost me $40 so it ought to be good looking. However, prices are so outrageous that $35 ready-made suits are shoddy. It is strictly tailored, the latest thing. My hat is a large black sailor, stylist, $5.00

Last night Mr and Mrs Perry and I went to the Alexandra to see "The Flame"—a very striking spectacular drama. It was a treat to get out. I like the Perrys very much. It is such a relief to know that you have been taking iron pills with advantage. I hope that you will continue to take the best of care of yourselves.

Now that Easter has come I suppose studies will cease at the Rectory. I have not much patience with those content to drift and play. There is too much to be done—and the doing is so interesting.

Certainly news from overseas is most encouraging and Kitchener's prophecy may be fulfilled. The Canadian part at Arras has been magnificent and surely it is a great support to know that the USA stand shoulder to shoulder with the Allies. Is Lee still in England? I am glad Alice and

Lev have had the comfort of his being there so long.

Heaps of love, have little to write about, my days consist of sleeps, milk diet and baths. Jane.

A month later, Pauline is officially on her way. Having joined up in Toronto she visited her parents in Centreville on her way to Halifax for embarkation. Her train trip took her to Saint John, where a stay-over allowed her time to be visited by cousins and her brother Guy (born 1873). The remainder of her journey turned out to be much more eventful. As she humorously relates to her parents, her colourful pale-blue CAMC nurse's uniform with red piping and brass buttons attracted the attention of rail officials. The train conductor and staff had been much distressed and anxious over a passenger who went into labour until they saw Pauline. Nursing Sister Balloch was soon in charge.

May 24, 1917

My Dearest Ones,

Of course you are awaiting a more detailed account of my adventures—cards are a limited medium though better than nothing at all. Ones' mind is so active and there is always so much to say—yet so many things (feelings, particularly) are "unwriteable."

You certainly sent me off like a soldier and I do not think you are going to regret letting me go. I cannot be thankful enough to Dr Peppers for taking us to Florenceville. It kept us together as long as possible and those were infinitely precious moments. I find many people anticipating the collapse of Germany at an early date and it may be that I shall not be away for a very long time after all—and a year soon rolls around. Have not the past six months seemed short indeed? The thing of importance to my mind is that you take most watchful care of yourselves—not exposing yourselves to the elements or the changes of atmosphere unprotected and not allowing slight indispositions to grow strong through neglect.

I am not anticipating trouble. After all I do have a sense of a divine providence—otherwise I would have been too great a coward to have continued on my present mission, for I have indeed been sorely tempted to turn back. To do so would be to shame you.

My train pulled into St John about 10:30 p.m. Rachael and Cort were there, Guy and Kath on the way. The two laggards appeared about 15 minutes later but fortunately the train was delayed, in fact, we did not pull out of St John until 4 a.m. so the cousins stayed with me...[until] 12 a.m. when I succeeded in sending them off and returned to my berth laden with parcels with which their loving thoughtfulness provided me.

K had for me a fountain pen, G a book—"father Fritz" as K calls him, a box of sweets, R a diary—(a line a day) which I mean to use and hope you will enjoy a year hence—if I am not on my way home by then I will send it. Cort gave me another box of sweets—both of which I am hoarding for consumption on ship board. Were they not kind? Guy wanted me to try and get leave to return for a day to St John—saying he would pay my fair if I only would ask. It was wonderfully good of him and he urged me so persistently that I would accept were it possible. However, we may sail before Sunday, without doubt very soon.

Our train was so many hours late that we did not pull into H [Halifax] until 3 p.m. but pray do not think the journey uneventful. As usual, the grey day took on considerable colour before its close, and twas my uniform that did it. Now it might be well for you to read the following lines each to yourself—and be prepared for a shock. It was about 10 a.m. when two conductors, one from the day coach and ours, appeared in excited consultation at the extreme end of the car gradually drawing near my section. Their faces expressed consternation and such phrases as "she said she won't get off" and "you will have to bring her in here and give her a section" and "get a doctor" reached my ears, and then one of them espied my uniform; his expression became carefree—jubilant. There followed whisperings and noddings and I was caught…[V]ery soon I found myself being ushered without protest conspicuously to the day coach to a woman with pinched white face who had been waiting her time since 11 p.m. the previous evening and had with her pure little "miniatures" all her own. She was bound for Londonderry. I escorted her back to the tourist car where she was given the stateroom, but determined to give her a little sound advice before assuming a doctor's office and thanks be—succeeded in convincing her that the only place of safety for her was a hospital. We were just pulling into Amherst and escorted by the kind hearted and intensely excited conductor and myself she took her departure from the train and was hurried off in an automobile to the hospital; and still very much in the public eye, with red trimmings and brass buttons shouting my profession, I returned thankfully to the comparative obscurity of my chair. Her small family was taken to Londonderry and there disposed of.

So much for adventure # 1. What next? but having heaps of fun? How about, arriving at the hospital where I reported and I found Kate Brown,[15] who may go over with me, then she too comes to this hotel.

It is a wet day so I may stay in and write letters, but I am Oh so thankful to be my own mistress until we sail. I shall try to make my letters as complete as possible and hope the boys many have the reading of them, though I shall write them, of course, too.

I was sorry not to have seen Marion at St John, but of course she could not get away at that hour.

Heaps of love to everybody; to Aunt Cass and Wilmot and more than I can ever tell to you, Paul.

Four days later and still in Halifax, Pauline writes her parents again.

15 Katherine L. Brown, born in Woodstock, New Brunswick, 1881; enlisted in the CAMC on April 26, 1917. She served in hospitals in Halifax and England.

She speaks of a shift in the Halifax Military Hospital, of friends she has met, and of which ship she may be sailing on. One possibility was the Olympic*—a sister ship to the* Titanic*—which was pressed into service as a troop transport at the beginning of the war due to its size and great speed. The key phrase in this letter, however, is Pauline's characterization of her state of mind as being "very optimistic and happy about my adventure." Such an upbeat statement could have been made by the men of the First Contingent like E. A. Poole in the early autumn of 1914, but to hear it in mid-1917 is striking indeed. Future correspondence will reveal if she retains this early enthusiasm.*

May 28, 1917

Dear Father and Mother,

When this reaches you I will be aboard ship, though perhaps still in harbour. It is not known upon which ship we sail though, the Olympic is at the pier and is said to be about to leave with troops—also the Letitia, a hospital ship which may carry 90 nurses.

At any rate it's little matter how we go, the chief thing is to get off now that we are en route. The Toronto draft are expected in this p.m., actually we have been expecting them since yesterday a.m. so they may arrive at the last minute in which case I shan't be able to have my cheques exchanged here but will have to wait. Thanks to the help in money dad gave me I have had sufficient for my needs—expenses here are $3.00 per day—exorbitant, but there was nothing else to do.

There must be a considerable sum coming to me and I shall send whatever I can spare. Have had lovely letters from Ottawa and have received yours. Hope my cards and letters have found you. Address me; Nursing Sister P. N. Balloch CAMC c/o Matron in Chief Macdonald 86 Stacek

Cecil Chambers, London, England. I am so glad to have an address to give you and perhaps I shall find a letter waiting for me. I have had such a pleasant time here with Miss Marian Jack—she is Sterling Jack's daughter—Mrs Bough, who is bound for Bermuda, where her soldier husband awaits her, and Miss Nichols of N.Y. Mrs Bough is delightful, very English and full of fun. I hope I shall meet them all again someday. Yesterday I was on duty at the Military Hosp. from 2 p.m. to 6:30 p.m. It was rather a farce, but I was simply being kept busy. This morning I was there again for a short while, but have the afternoon free. Will walk out after this letter is written. Have walked around the park and think I shall "do" the Gardens this p.m.

Went to St Paul's yesterday a.m. I listened to Dr Armitage, a dear old man and stayed to Communion. It had greater significance than usual for me. I sent several cards from here; one to Dr Peppers and one to Bessie Campbell. They were kind. I am very optimistic and happy about my adventure. I feel sure that nothing but good can come from it, and you have been and will be a wonderful help to me. I am enclosing a letter for Mary, she understands so much. I am also sending the book Guy gave me and which I have enjoyed.

Your daughter Jane.

A hasty note scribbled the next morning announced that she was finally leaving Canada.

May 29

Peep o'day,

I awoke to the song of tug-boats chug-chug, chug-chug and knew that today is the day. I am to be at the pier at 10 a.m., that means 9:45 a.m. for I shall be there on time!

Have not yet seen any of the Toronto nurses. They may have come last night (when they were expected) and they may have been carried direct to the boat. Last night soldiers were going aboard in sheaves they say.

Mrs Bough and I walked to the citadel late yesterday afternoon and looked down on the city from all sides, glorified by distance and sunlight. I was so fortunate as to meet her on my return from the Public Gardens, where I had been strolling. I had my $15 remaining exchanged for pound notes so I will have some English "coin" if I need it.

I had hoped my $150 would come to me in time to be mailed to Guy from here. Will have to write about that later. I owe him $3.15 and Mary $6.00 for materials for underwear.

Love to all my village friends, particularly Alice Mildred and Mrs Jack Lee, Love Paul.

A letter Pauline received from a former patient before she left sheds some light on Pauline's personality and skills. The two apparently had shared much in their time together, and this young woman writes of both Pauline's relationship with her parents and her nursing skills.

May 20, 1917
Ottawa

Dear Pauline,

Just now the ordeal of parting with your dearest on earth is taking place and you all are suffering as keenly as though the pang were a physical one. Love and friendship however are spiritual and continue though sundered far apart. I know your unselfish parents have made it as easy for you as possible, but one cannot entirely hide emotion on such occasions.

It is so splendid a thing for you to be going and I know it will mean blessing, comfort and succour to many, many a poor sufferer. Do I not know what an immeasurable help you are when fighting for life? and the comfort you gave me I could not have had even from my husband, who would have given the world to lessen the anguish of those awful days.

Pauline arrived in England on June 9 and her "adventure" continued. Her friendship with a young nursing sister, Dorothy M. Baldwin[16] of Toronto, proved immediately beneficial. Though born in Paris, Ontario, Miss Baldwin had well-to-do English relatives who took both her and Pauline under their wing. These English relatives gave the two women a London base for their travels and the chance to stay at an elegant country estate. Clearly, they enjoyed their week's rest before commencing their duties. The ladies shopped in London, toured Westminster Abbey, Bushy Park, Hampton Court, and Kew Gardens. They had hot baths both before bed and first thing in the morning, drank tea in bed before rising, and ate strawberries dipped in thick cream and frosted with sugar. Needless to say, these were luxuries they would not be enjoying as nursing sisters in the hospitals.

Rosebank, Angel Hill, Sutton, Surrey, England,
June 13, 1917

16 D. M. Baldwin, born 1891, daughter of Robert and Mary Baldwin of Paris, Ontario.

Does not the above suggest all loveliness and peace and to think that I should be in such a spot? It is all because of my friendship for Dorothy Baldwin—a most fortunate thing for me, though it is comforting to know that her aunt in Canada and her people here seem to be very glad of our attachment to each other.

You have read of our adventures up to Sunday evening. Monday morning we rested but immediately after luncheon came to Sutton and there were met by Miss Robinson who took us with her to Belmont to her brother's house. He has just recently returned from India where he had been for over 20 years, giving up his place (he himself is not in physical condition) though here he goes on military police duty daily. We had delicious tea and a long talk, in the course of which delightful things were planned for us and Miss R insisted that I come back with Dorothy to stay the rest of the week. We went home early and straight to bed for we had busy plans for Tuesday. Tuesday morning we shopped. Dorothy had to get a regulation item of clothing and we needed a few small articles. We know so little of London that we waste time going about on busses so we invariably take a taxi and go direct. Dorothy had a letter of introduction to Mr Cyril Cassel, manager of the Bank of Montreal, Threadwell Street, so down we went. We had a very gratifying interview (he was most kind), deposited our checks and reserved 10£ for present needs.

June 14: Left off rather abruptly to have a full day, which I shall try to do justice to with my pen in due course of time. After luncheon on Tuesday, we paid our bill at the Kingsley, took a taxi to Victoria Station where we left our club bags and then went to Westminster Abbey where our uniforms got for us a seat in the choir, where we enjoyed a lovely anthem and heard Sir Henry Bridges, the organist. After the service, we engaged a guide to take us through the Abbey. Many wonderful things have been removed; parts of the oldest and most famous tombs, lovely windows, the removal and replacing of each will cost 300 or 400 £ (fancy what their value must be) but there were two wonderful rose windows for us to look at and many tombs that were not completely hidden by sand bags—

the poets corner, the chapel where King George has his official chair and opposite, the Duke of Connaught, and down below seats on which the monks sat made in some clever fashion so that if by chance a weary old fellow should fall asleep up would go the seat and he would fall off so they were called miserere seats. We saw the coronation chair and where the chair is placed at the great ceremony, and where the king and queen take their places, also the great lords and ladies and bishops—not a very great number can witness the event, also Wolfe's monument draped with the banners of Canadian battalions. Also effigies of Queen Elizabeth, Nelson, Charles II and other monarchs—each made at the time of the death of said person, dressed in the clothes last worn by him and carried before his body at the funeral. They are under glass and very well preserved. We went through so quickly and saw so much that I cannot give you a very clear impression of what we saw.

We had just time to catch the 5:22 train at Victoria Station and came to Sutton where we were met by Mrs Bliss, a sister of Miss Robinson, who brought us here and where we received the kindest of welcomes. I cannot tell you how lovely Miss R has been to me, a stranger and that Dorothy, who has such lovely connections in England, should be fond of me and insist on having me with her always is unheard of good fortune. If being her friend can repay her in the least I shall do my utmost. She has just finished her training and lacks experience so I may be of use to her. Well, we had a delicious and satisfactory supper, then a walk in the garden, then a hot bath and bed. And such a sleep as we had! to wake up next morning to a cup of tea at our bed before rising, then another bath and breakfast. This is the loveliest spot. I cannot do it justice—but the name Rosebank, Angel Hill speaks volumes. At present we are sitting under a rose bower in a garden of roses; pink, red and creamy, with ivy climbing over the walls, with lilies, delphinium and other flowers all about. Just across from our bedroom windows is the church, cobblestone, ivy covered, wonderful oaks and elms—a dream realized. We are having exceptional weather, sunny and warm. Today the first cloud, but it is passing.

To resume my story; after breakfast Miss Robinson had Letherford, the housekeeper, put up a lunch of sandwiches and cakes and off we went to Hampton Court to spend the day. We went by train to Wimbledon and there took a tram to Kingston through a veritable garden at Kingston we quickly found Bushy Park, the most wonderful English park your imagination can picture, long broad avenues of ancient chestnuts…, deer, a great fountain and pond, with lilies and swans in the centre of an enormous circular lawn surrounded by magnificent trees, with wide alluring paths leading into misty, obscure distances. One's fancy took strange flight and peopled the lovely scene with lords and ladies of long ago. Here we refreshed ourselves with sandwiches and water and then we left the Park and entered the grounds of Hampton Court. First, we were told we must enter "the Maze" and Miss R. had provided herself with a book lest we should be a long time finding our way out. We entered through a grey gate and started off to the left between tall hedges, on we went winding about, doubling back, circling and sometimes finding ourselves at the end of a path. Fortunately, when we started out we took a certain house and tree as landmarks. At last we found ourselves at the centre where we sat down and rested on a bench—the keeper had called them chairs, and then we returned. We were not long getting back, greatly to the surprise of the gate keeper and Miss R. Then we walked through the loveliest garden of trees, vines and flowers. I must not fail to mention the copper birch, a lovely copper coloured tree. Then we came to a wide green lawn, with baths and wonderful beds of flowers and a fountain with water—blues, white and red and to our right, Hampton Court Palace. Miss R. waited outside for us and we went on to explore and came out with our eyes hanging on our cheeks. Now I cannot tell you where we went nor how, but I will try to give you some of my impressions. It is built around an inner court, where by the way the grass had been allowed to grow and was cut for hay and lay drying. We passed through and into the court and across to the other side. Just over the arch was a great clock, 24 hours dial, with curious signs and figures upon its face.

Inside we found a great stairway up which we were directed by a policeman, who, by the way saluted us, to the art galleries. Well, we walked and walked through rooms and chambers, large and small, hung with pictures and portraits, historical scenes, religious, allegorical and a few of flowers, giant tapestries, armour, weapons of all kinds arranged in conventional and artistic fashion upon the walls. Several of these rooms had been chambers of kings and queens, and there were still their beds with canopy tops and posts of beautiful wood—hung and covered with rather frayed materials of ye olden time. I must say I am glad we sleep on simple beds between clean sheets of white spread (I am not referring to my hospital ship cot). I would have exchanged it for a plank of the village sidewalk. Finally, we came to the room of Cardinal Wolsey, who by the way was the first to build the Palace, his fireplace and Henry's room. Then we came out, found Miss Robinson, went to see "The Vine," a wonderful grape vine 900 years old, the garden of Henry VIII, and then back to the gardens again. From here we walked to the Thames, found a little place where we had bread and butter and tea at an awful price and then took the boat down the river, past house boats, wonderful gardens, through two locks and under bridges, until after we passed Richmond Bridge we came to Kew Gardens. They were lovely, of course, a marvel, had we not just come from Bushy Park and Hampton Court.

The next day we dined at Belmont with Mrs Bliss, Miss Robinson's sister. There were strawberries, a basketful. We had luncheon, delicious, ending with great strawberries luscious and sweet, which were not hulled. We dipped them in sugar and thick cream. If you wish to taste heaven, try it. We stayed for afternoon tea, then home. Tonight we two had dinner alone and now are writing in the garden while our fairy godmother is away on some other heavenly mission.

We are both so happy and enjoying the precious privilege of this sweet visit here. On Sunday we will be on duty at Orpington. Meanwhile there are wonderful plans for us tomorrow and Saturday. Could old friends be kinder?

Heaps of love and send this on to my dear brothers and sisters—they will return to you, daughter, P.

As planned, Nursing Sisters Balloch and Baldwin reported to Ontario Military Hospital at Orpington in Kent on Saturday evening, June 16. Duty commenced the next day, and the transition from being so extensively pampered to the grind of routine daily duty was not an easy one. In her letter to her parents, Pauline does not dwell on her work, for so much of her adventures in London remained to be related. Her grand experience included a trip to London Bridge, Fishmongers' Hall, St. Dunstan's Church, Tower Bridge, and the Tower of London, St. Paul's, and Kensington Gardens, not to mention lobsters for dinner and, of course, those strawberries dipped in cream topped with sugar!

June 17, 1917
Ontario Military Hospital, Orpington, Kent Co., England

Dear Father and Mother,

Dorothy and I reached here last night about 8:30 p.m. expecting to go on duty this a.m. and the expected happened. It was none too easy. The thought of hard work after the luxurious time that has been ours. I found a letter from Lee waiting for me and we are going to try to have an afternoon together, perhaps in London. It will be lovely for both of us, also this morning a letter from Miss Fowlds, a Toronto acquaintance, perhaps I should say friend; but so far nothing from home. However, I am not disappointed for I have expected nothing knowing how long it takes for mail to come, but I do hope that mine to you are not dallying on the way.

Now I must give you a history of the remainder of my visit at Sutton, for it was so delightful and I want you to share my pleasure in so far as you may. On Thursday morning we were awakened in the usual lovely way by Miss Robinson with a cup of tea and roses, and at 10 a.m. were met at the station by Mr Fred Robinson who had a day of sightseeing in London planned for us. I can't begin to do the day justice but will do my utmost. We got off the train at London Bridge, walked over the old bridge into old London. At the end of the bridge to the left is Fishmongers' Hall, an old and famous institution, the building now being used as a hospital. Just near the entrance was a great gun taken from the Boers at Pretoria and used by the English at Ladysmith; from here we walked to Billingsgate fish market, a huge, busy, crowded, shiny, smelly place where we saw fishes of all kinds, large and small, dead and alive, lobsters black, lobsters boiling, lobsters boiled, eels in casks, squirming to be cooked alive—no thank you! Coming out we looked on the Customs House, then took a side turning through a narrow street, up a hill, and saw the old church of St Dunstan's in the east. To get a view of its spire for which it is famous, we entered an office building and were taken in an elevator to the roof, from which we saw not only the famous spire, designed by the way, by the daughter of Sir Christopher Wren, but also Tower Bridge and much of old London. Nearby to the old church of All Hallows, across Tower Hill we saw Trinity House and the moat and then we visited the Tower. It was most interesting, from the gardens from which we again saw Tower Bridge, to the moat, now dry, old portcullis tower built by William II where the boy princes were imprisoned and murdered and known as the bloody tower, the old crypt and cells, the wall that is said to date from the time of Julius Caesar, though the tower was begun by the Conqueror, crown jewels and sceptre—imitations of course.

We had luncheon at "The Tavern." Then we saw a bit more of the old city of London and then took a bus and rode to St Paul's. From there to Hyde Park, on to Kensington Gardens, where we saw Kensington Palace where Queen Victoria was born, then we walked through the gardens to a cool shady place where we had tea and bread and cake—then walked down Kensington Street past Albert Memorial and Hall and finally took a bus ride through the city, the Pall Mall area and on to the station. We came back to Miss Robinson's very weary but very happy. She had a delicious supper for us, lobster (fresh) and delicious strawberries. You must try them on the stem with very thick cream and sugar. Put a spoonful of sugar at the side of your plate and pour on it a little cream. Then dip the strawberry in it, Yum!! We were weary after such a long day of course, so took hot baths and went to bed. We had our breakfast in bed next morning and each day bloomed with a red, red rose. Then we visited a friend's rose garden—a marvel of blooms, had luncheon, spent a restful afternoon and in the evening came here.

I cannot tell you how good Miss Robinson was. She made me as welcome as one of her own and has given me the freedom of her house. I am to go at any time just as Dorothy, she said she would mother us and she wishes us to come to her at any time for anything. I thanked her for her most kind generosity toward me and I left with a tear in my eye. I wish you would write a note—her address is Miss Robinson, Rosebank, Angel Hill, Sutton, Surrey, England.

I forgot to tell you that Miss R., in the course of our day in London, insisted in giving us each a beautiful pair of tan gloves. We had some photographs taken about $2.00 a dozen—very good I think. We will give the Robinsons and Mrs Bliss each one as souvenirs and the rest I shall probably send to you, one for each of the boys, one for Col and Mrs Carrick, unless you have sent one of the others—address Port Arthurs, and keep the others until you hear from me about them. I hope you are both well and enjoying the lovely summer. Don't worry about me, there is no reason.

Paul

Although her particular hospital wing was not yet open, by late June Pauline was settled into a routine and regular nursing work at the hospital in Orpington. She relates her respect and perhaps even awe for her matron who, having served in France was, not surprisingly, a strong and distinct personality. She tells of a trip through the beautiful Kentish countryside, but the reality of war is also present. She remarks on treatments designed to "bring misshapen and helpless limbs back to something of their old efficiency" and of the "repairs that are done on soldiers' poor marred faces and limbs." Even her trip through the countryside to Ramsgate in search of her cousin "Rainie"[17] *is an occasion to relate bombing damage caused by a German Zeppelin air raid. Unfortunately, Pauline missed Rainie. As she discovers, he was already on his way back to Canada. Rainie's case was both tragic and sad. A victim of "shell shock," his service file reveals a man who, despite treatment, remained seriously impaired. Attempts to find him useful employment at bases in England also failed. Finally, the army discharged him, and he returned to Canada in August 1917. His family must have found him a very different man from the person they had so proudly sent to war.*

Ontario Military Hospital, Orpington, England
June 23

Dear Father and Mother,

Nearly a month since I left Canada and quite that since I left home and still the long silence to be bridged by a letter. It's not a long wait and I realize an unavoidable one so I am not anxious, yet I hope you have been receiving my letters and cards for some time.

17 Douglas Rainsford Balloch (424541), born in Edmundston, New Brunswick, and married to Florence Bachan Balloch.

We are having such wonderful weather for England, no rain until yesterday. The work here is very light, too light to be interesting, but 60 of the new sisters (there were 90 of us who came on the Letitia) were sent to Orpington. From there, some who were already here and some of us may be sent to France, but it will not be immediately. Meanwhile, I spend most of my time here on duty in the new wing where there are, as yet, no patients, and which will not be opened until July 5. We have been counting, marking and arranging linens; making beds, lecturing to orderlies, gleaning what information we can concerning Military Hospital routine and etiquette. Then enjoying from three to four hours daily off duty and sometimes more. It takes time to adjust and to place advantageously so many new nurses but I shall be very glad to get at real work though no doubt this preparation, while slow, is necessary.

The sisters here are very fine, many of them have seen active service for two and more years in France. They are broad-minded, interesting women whom one cannot help respecting and liking. Miss Carstairs who is in charge of the new section is one of these and I find her fascinating. Her appearance is most unusual and interesting—tall, slight, moderately thin long oval face, fine brown eyes, with well marked brow, (expression, indescribable; so many possibilities) very high, thin nose and large, well shaped mouth, slightly smiling. I like to look at her all the time, she looks an enigma, and I believe she is one. It is delightful to meet someone who is not commonplace; most of us are duplicates to be seen in every town and every country.

On Wednesday I was given the day to go to Ramsgate to see Rainie. It happened to be a fruitless errand as he had been sent away to Canada, I think, as there was some comfort to take the sharp edge off the disappointment. I so wanted to write Aunt Celia and Flo that I had seen him but now they do not need the comfort of a letter of that sort since they have him with them. It was a wonderful trip down, such country, through Kent you know. It is wonderful to have these glimpses of England. It was not much level country in Surrey, more undulating though there were great level stretches. I would like to talk of it to Mr Scholey. I know he has a mental picture of what I have seen; lovely orchards, great fields of hops, symmetrical rows, quaint, brick stone and "plaster" houses—with curious looking buildings nearby, with cone-shaped tops, where I bet the hops are dried—old stone churches and then presently the [Medway]—widening gradually, with what looked like marsh land along its banks and sailing boats with terra cotta sails and here and there tiny streams so quiet and level they looked like canals, and then the distance not clear like ours, but an atmosphere that looked as though by stretching out your hand it might be touched. That may have been a herald of the rain that came later on. At last we came to Ramsgate harbour. It was only a short way to the hospital so I walked from the station, past some wharfs where a few days before the Germans had dropped bombs, destroying buildings into a narrow street or lane, then up winding stone steps to the street above (all the windows in the buildings shattered by the shock of explosions). The hospital was at one time a hotel but it had been converted into a very well equipped hospital for wounded soldiers, electrical treatment, baths, violet rays, massage—and so on, everything to bring misshapened and helpless limbs back to something of their old efficiency. I could find no trace of Rainie, though everybody was most kind. Finally, an officer directed me to the Princess Patricia Hospital. He was not there but the sisters did all they could to locate him by telephone communication with other hospitals; there are several there, and at last I was told that his name had been on the list of those for transfer to Canada. I am hoping there is no mistake. Just before I left it rained in torrents but cleared when we boarded the train. I say we, for one of the nursing sisters, who had been in France, came with me. It was wonderful to watch the sun breaking through the heavy clouds, to see the brightness of its light on field and trees in contrast to black shadows underneath—and then a rainbow. I think I told you how luxurious is the foliage here, the green so dense, I got into Victoria Station London about 7 p.m. and as I had only 20 minutes decided not to get any refreshment until I reached

Orpington, which happened at 8:30. I was very hungry and knew it was quite late to get anything at the house so tried the village but found every place closed. Finally, as I had quite made up my mind to go dinnerless to bed, I passed a cosy cottage with Grange House over the door and a young woman in the door way talking to a soldier and I think the young woman of the house must have suggested hospitality for after a moment's hesitation, I turned back and asked if it would be possible to get some refreshment there. She said certainly and brought me in, explaining that the mistress of the house did serve meals but that she and her mother occupied two rooms and were just to have dinner and insisted on sharing theirs. Protests were vain and I stayed, enjoying my adventure very much. They were delightful people—good looking and charming manners—Cavell, the name, the daughter a frequent visitor to the hospital here. She sent by me a great armful of flowers to a patient whose army chum was to be buried next day. He and his bedside neighbour made a beautiful cross with the flowers and their gratitude was touching. They are such interesting fellows for the most part, even turning to embroidery to keep themselves amused and they embroider well, often copying the badge of their battalion in silks or wool. It's so wonderful, the repairs that are done on their poor marred faces and limbs and they are all so patient and optimistic.

I am going to write Lee soon and see if we can have some time together and will try to get in touch with Fred Gordon. I think they would like to see somebody fresh from home.

Had a letter from Uncle Charlie last night which I shall answer tonight. He may be able to have me placed with him. It was good to hear. Also heard from Mrs Fitz-Randolph at Oxford—asking me for a weekend. Kind of her but I know it cannot be arranged now. Baldie (Nursing Sister Baldwin or Dorothy) has just brought me another letter from Uncle Chas, such a lovely one. If he can have us taken on together in the Boulogne hospital No. 3 Canadian General—we shall be very glad. She is a dear and much younger than I, and I think we are very good for each other.

Someday when I write I shall try to describe this hospital but I want to know a little more about it first. Of course you are sharing my letters with the "children." Must write Guy tonight or in the morning but he understands that these are joint letters. Love to all my friends.

Hope they will treat me to a line now and again.

Heaps of love, Daughter. Take good care of yourselves.

Note the change in title of the letter below. Pauline had heard from home, and it moves her to address her mother most intimately. She was very close to her parents, and it grieved her that they worried about her so. They were then relatively healthy, but if that were to change she would drop all and return home. Her letter is not all serious; however, she relates the purchase of a bicycle and the wondrous trips she and her friend Dorothy made through the surrounding English countryside. The Uncle Charlie she mentions appears to be Captain Charles G. Main, who was married to Pauline's cousin Caroline May (Balloch). Charles, born in St. Andrews, New Brunswick, joined the CAMC in April 1916 and was serving at a Canadian hospital in France.

July 4, 1917

Dearest Mommy,

Your letter came today, such a joy to me—don't ever say you are dull. What you write is always lovely and interesting, and as I write, I know you are feeling differently about me, less anxiety for you have had my cable and some of my letters and know that I have plenty to eat. Up to date I have had such a pleasant time, have seen such interesting sights with no hard work that I am almost forced to wonder why I was so strongly moved to come, and so bring such sorry to you.

Uncle Charlie writes me that work in France is slack too so our boys are not being destroyed as they were and one is deeply thankful for that. Some think that autumn will indeed bring us victory and if it does you will have me at home in the spring—not very far away. If you feel ill and need me, call—nothing could keep me here. On the other hand, I feel confident you will take good care of yourselves for my sake, which if you do, will ensure your wellbeing until I get home again, for organically you and dad are well, and if you do not expose yourselves to too great exertion and take care of yourselves when indisposed you should have many years still in which to give your children joy. I am really not so far away though it seems a great distance to you. I think there is no longer any danger of famine—restrictions on potatoes are off, an excellent sign.

I have a tremendous appetite and plenty of nourishing food. I seem to be no nearer the field of battle here than I did in Toronto. The nursing sister, like the soldier, is seen to thrive in this atmosphere, leading this life.

My bicycle was an extravagance but it makes getting about so easy, and is giving me glimpses of England that I should otherwise have to go without.

Monday night Dorothy and I rode above the hospital about a mile then made a turning to the right into a long narrow road, very like our own country roads, eventually we turned into a lane on our left, winding gradually up hill, not too steep, so that we were able to keep to our wheels, through lovely winding places, and then fields of oats or other grain and sometimes brilliant with poppies, up, up, up—rather lovely for the most part. Then coming unexpectedly upon a tower with a clock—not a church or hall, just a farmer's fancy for his house with outbuildings about, then on and on until we came to the loveliest hamlet. They say the loveliest in Kent, called Down, with an old stone church within a church yard, narrow winding streets. Then we circled about and returned by the high road, paved, without roughness and all the way down hill we coasted without putting foot to peddle for quite four miles and came at last to the point where we made the first turning to the left.

Last night we took another course and rode straight ahead all upgrade, but so gradual it seemed to be level. We coasted home with a lovely sunset in our faces, casting soft purple and rose light on windswept fields, ivy covered walls, gardens and trees, sheep folds, all lovely things that continue to make a perfect English landscape. It seems selfish to be enjoying so much when there is so much suffering and with you and dad at home with anxious heart.

I am so glad that you are to have aunt Celia and Jean. I hope they will stay long. To think that your birthday is here once more, how the years sprint around so quickly, it takes our breath. All my hearts to you tonight dear. Dorothy sends love and best wishes for many happy returns. She wants to know you, she is a sweet thing and deserves just such a treat some day.

Hope you are getting all my cards and letters, Daughter Jane.

Exciting news: Pauline is going to France! Her destination will be No. 3 Canadian Stationary Hospital (CSH) at Doullens, midway between Amiens and Arras. Her excitement and joy come across very clearly in this letter to her mother. Although they might worry that she is closer to real danger, Pauline cannot contain her childlike enthusiasm at being sent to the continent. From now on she will be able to write on the outside of the envelopes to her parents: "on active duty."

July 25, 1917
Kingsley Hotel, London

Dear Mother,

I am at the Kingsley for luncheon, then heigh ho for Folkestone en route for France—No 3 Stationary Hospital. Address letters as usual. I know you will be interested in these awful snaps—my Kodak will be of no use to me in France—taboo!, but on leave will be a great pleasure. Heaps of love and don't worry. I'm just beginning to live. A scurvy Airedale pup adopted Baldie and me yesterday and escorted us to the station at Orpington today. Great luck—we are sorry to leave our mascot behind.

Daughter Jane

It is as if she could read her parents' minds! She is certain they are now more worried about her than before. Yes, she is in France, and yes, it rains constantly and she lives in a tent, but they know how she loves the outdoors life. Above all, she is content. At present, her clothes are sufficient, but she asks for colder-weather supplies, for winter will surely come. She would tell more, but where she is censorship is strict. Her boss, Matron Miss Wilson, has put Pauline in charge of the kitchen and dining room, a new position which means no direct nursing but which involves a learning curve and much new responsibility.

August 1, 1917
France

Dear Father and Mother,

First and foremost to set your dear hearts at rest, I am well and happy and not overworked. If you could see me as I am and conditions about me you would have no further anxiety about me and except for the loneliness you feel at times because of my absence, you would be quite happy about me.

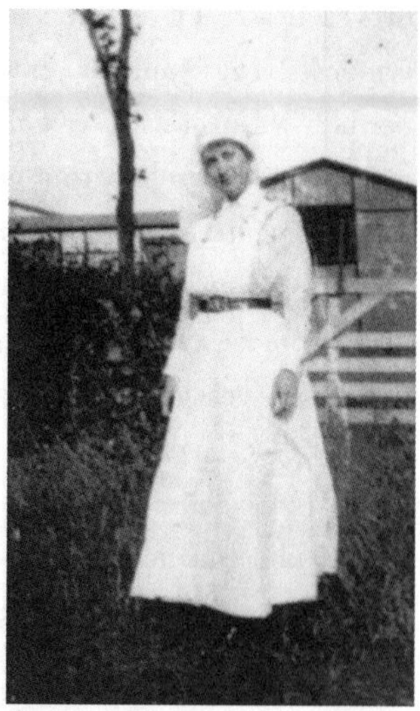

Pauline on break.

Unfortunately, I cannot tell you all I see and hear and do—not that doing so would, in my case do any harm, but I am where the censorship is most strict and not any chances are taken. I have never felt or looked better and shall take good care of myself. So cease to worry about me, like dears, I hate to cause you anxiety and if only you could know the little need there is of that! Frankly, I am much better off than I was for I am content.

It has rained persistently since we came, such a change from the summer months in England. Yesterday we took a long walk in the wet lands in rubber from head to heel and returned with our arms full of poppies. Today Miss Wilson, the matron, came to our section and left instructions that I be put in charge of the kitchen and dining rooms—a new post and why she chose such a green horn as myself I do not know. However, I take the plunge tomorrow. It means considerable responsibility. At any rate I shall be learning something. There will be no nursing for me at present and that I truly regret for my heart is in it always. If a fine day would only come I would make a sketch of our tent. We have plenty of room and are as cosy as can be. We have a small oil stove and can heat water. Matting is stretched from one end to the other and a screen separates our end from Mrs McLean's. I love it. It is a great improvement on stone walls, doors and windows. The simple life, but very comfortable. You have only to remember how enthusiastic I have always been about tenting and life in the open generally to know how thoroughly I enjoy this.

I have written only one other letter from here. I hope it reached you. In it I spoke of woollen underwear, meaning the things I would like for winter. I have an excellent supply of shoes but my boots are so large that in the cold weather I mean to wear two pairs of socks, cashmere and then knitted stockings outside of them. I have woollen bloomers and corset covers but want a flannel petticoat and will be glad of a little hug-me-tight—blue like my uniforms. Don't knit these things mother, have the things and jacket knitted for me. I am going to send to England for a pair of blankets to sleep between when the cooler weather comes. I am taking no chance you see! Now confess, this is a rosy rose letter, I repeat, lest the other failed to reach you. Must have a nap and then back to duty. Remember me to everybody.

Heaps and heaps of love, Polly, How is Jane? I never could abide her.

Pauline's excitement has not waned. She is safe, she is content, and she is well, but she has a problem. She realizes that the more she tells her parents of her well-being and contentment, the more it may have the opposite effect of stimulating them to think that her reassurances are overcompensation for a truly awful situation. So she turns her attention to describing her patients. They are mostly young men—meaning in their early to mid-twenties—and, in her hospital, all officers. Tellingly, by this stage of the war, many of them had become commissioned by rising from the ranks. They occupy their hours by drawing or sketching. One man constantly polishes his pipe. Pauline does not yet reflect that the man's fixation with his pipe might indicate deeper, unsettling psychological issues.

August 6, 1917
3rd Canadian Stationary Hospital, BEF, France

Dearest Mum and Dearest Dad,

How does it feel to have your first, last and only daughter "somewhere in France"? I cannot hope to let you know just how comfortable and happy I am until I get home. You will always think there are deprivations and dangers and exposures. I fear that by constantly insisting that I have plenty to eat, of good and wholesome things, comfortable bed, plenty of sleep, walks, and time for resting, will fail to convince you of my wellbeing and yet such is the unromantic fact. I never was in better physical condition or better content. I got your letter today, also one from Mary written from Jersey City and one from Mrs Dennis, a beautiful note that I shall treasure always, and in a day or two shall send to you to keep for me. I know you will enjoy it, though I don't deserve such praise, but realize that her feeling for me is coloured by my association with Mary. She is a very wonderful old lady, the loveliest I have known, always excepting my mother and I shall always feel knowing her to have been an unusual privilege.

Baldie [Dorothy] has had several letters from her brother[18] who is not far from here and she expects to be able to see him. I hope they will be able to meet, I have no idea where Lee White is but shall try again to get in touch with him for if he is anywhere within reach I want to see him and if far away I can write and send him little things.

I am finding things easy so far and very pleasant. I am on the officers wards and like them. Most of them are very young, just two or three older men, and they are dears—the young chaps of course I mean. It is quite astonishing, the things they can do—two of them sketch well and a third, an older man, daubs for the sake of something to do, makes very interesting sketches, though not at all beautiful. Some of them play well, and can bring quite unusual music out of the old organ that they have at their disposal. One of them, who is still in bed, and reads constantly, is a lover of the weed, and treats his pipe with great absorption. I frequently find him polishing the bowl of his briar pipe until now it is a lovely mahogany hue and beautiful lustre. Today he asked me for a bit of silk and was delighted when I brought it to him. He is a quiet chap, but interesting.

Another who has just gone, is a Lieutenant in the Lancashire Light Infantry, has risen from the ranks, has been decorated with the Military Cross and is overflowing with zip. He is Irish and adorable—hollers when excited and had very bright brown eyes.

We have two others of the [Royal Flying Corps] and [Australian Flying Corps]—the latter Australian infantry men, in the ranks at first and

18 Although born in England, Dorothy's brother was in the Australian infantry.

then transferred. We shall lose them soon and will miss them too. They'll be off to the north where there is heavy fighting.

I got some postal cards down town today but hardly think I will send them. I will try one later. If it gets through, let me know. There is no reason why they shouldn't pass. Now I must sleep. My thoughts are home, night and morning and many times daily.

Pauline

Although she does not have much to write about, Pauline dashes off a short note concerning their tent. She and Baldie have decided to decorate their little living quarters. What is really just a tent to sleep in has also to serve as a daytime sitting area, and the women exercise great ingenuity in accomplishing the transformation.

August 10, 1917
No. 3 Canadian Stationary Hospital

Dearest Ones,

I have little new to write tonight. Baldie and I have been covering boxes arranged for bureaus with chintz that I bought from London, also a table that serves as a wash stand (oil cloth on top, and objectionable items out of sight underneath) and the camp chair. We are going to buy something bright on which to cover our pillows for day time use and to hang as curtains to separate our half of the hut from the other. The cretonne I bought has a background of white lattice and blue and lavender flower design, with suggestions of yellow to warm it—very striking, artistic, and serviceable. It harmonizes very nicely with our puffs which we got in England; ground and border, blue with sufficient suggestion of red to give warmth. My trunk serves as a settee and by day is covered with my warm rug and made inviting with my blue pillow. It is really very attractive. I am enclosing a postal card which I am sure will be allowed to pass. Please let me know if you receive it. I am sending a letter to Jack in the same mail. Have had most, if not all of your letters. They are my delight. Hope you are as well as I. I cannot wish you better than that.

Oceans of love, "Daughter Jane"

The same day, Pauline pens a more serious letter to her father. She tells him of interesting walks, of discovering a château, of her "fame" as a sketch artist, and of the large roadside crucifixes which were commonplace in Flanders. She is adamant that she will not harp on about how well she is doing and how content she is, for that would be redundant. Amazingly, she then concludes by telling her father that she has had her locket engraved with her name and rank—a measure infinitely preferable to the identification disc that were issued to all ranks so that human remains could be correctly identified.

August 10, 1917
No. 3 Canadian Stationary Hospital, BEF, France

Dear Dad,

I had your lovely long letter today; such a pleasure telling me that my letters are finding you with little delay and I am so glad and it means so much to me to know that you are not too lonely. Surely it would not have done for me to have remained idle at home or doing useless things in Toronto with such opportunity for service on this side of the water.

It's so true and you must be comforted by and happy in the knowledge that nurses here are greatly considered and well cared for and so far I have not been overworked. On the contrary, I think all my letters of late have contained such comforting assurance so I shall not repeat myself again for some time.

Just think of me as in the pink of condition, working about nine hours a day with one afternoon and half of Sunday off each week. I am having interesting talks with men who are taking a well earned rest from serious strain and arduous tasks, some recovering from ills. When off duty I am taking walks along roads, planked by symmetrical rows of trees or through interesting villages or the streets of this town, walking on cobble stones, to which my feet are gradually becoming accustomed, or through mud with which they are more or less familiar.

Today I bought a walking stick for two francs, twenty-five centimes, about 45¢ and thoroughly enjoyed using it. I have congratulated myself many times that I brought my colours. Some of my patients draw very well and we have been exchanging ideas on paper. One awfully nice chap of the Royal Flying Corps came to me the other day and asked me to sketch him. I felt in the mood and made an attempt which everyone said was a likeness and it must have been for it was recognized by several who had not seen me at work on it. I became famous at once as a portrait painter. Since then we have all been daubing madly and if I grant all requests for souvenirs from my brush I will be an excessively busy woman. I painted a sister today against a background of green, for a nice, middle aged captain and he was genuinely delighted. It was nice of him to be so pleased for it was really quite a daub, though I caught a sweet expression.

I am delighted that you are so pleased with the photographs. I thought the proofs so dreadful that I had some more taken in England, an extravagance, but I wanted you to have something better than they promised to be. I am going to send one to uncle Charlie who is very anxious to have one, so don't send one of these to Aunt Case for she can share yours with you. I am glad aunt Celia's has her boys with her. I was thoroughly disappointed not to have seen Rainie.

I hope both Frank and Rainie have made the best of recoveries and that I shall see Guy in France.

PAULINE D. BALLOCH

Dorothy and I had a p.m. today. We had some tennis (I did not play for I loathe chasing balls), and sat talking to two charming boys convalescing—they would hate being called boys. After dinner D. and I walked to a village about I I/4 miles from here and through the most wonderful park onto an old French Chateau. We found our way by paths along a quiet street through gates, up a steep hill (aided by our treasured walking sticks) to a lovely road bordered by magnificent smooth barked trees, which we followed for nearly I/4 mile until we came to great iron gates. The gates being closed, we came back a short distance and forced an opening on to the highway through the hedges. We were at the top of a hill looking back at a glorious sunset shining on the little village in the valley and away to the east fields of wheat that had been cut and stacked with here and there a peasant out of one of Millet's masterpieces. The beautiful fields of unripe oats, with here and there a white plaster and brick farm house and black and green trees against a sky of vivid blue with streaky clouds the wind had left. Now and again we passed a peasant with heavy horses of the Ross Bonus type resting by the roadside or a man driving in an awkward looking dogcart with "buggy" top. At the junction of the road with the one that brought us home was a lovely grove of trees with a lawn in the centre. We went in and there was a crucifix—almost life-sized. They are to be seen very frequently in France and one of the English officers, not a Romanist, was telling me that they all observed, no matter how great the destruction round about, these monuments always seem to escape, as if they are especially protected.

I hope to hear where Lee is soon—also Frank Goring and Rod Maclauchlin. Had a letter today from Guy—such an interesting one. I will write him soon. Hope all is as well with you as with me. More, I cannot wish anyone. I had my locket engraved with my name N.S. C.A.M.C. instead of an identification disc. It is a great comfort to me having your picture.

Your loving daughter, Pauline.

Although she claims to have "so little to say," her letter of late August brims with news: letters received, entertaining concerts, interesting patients, and delightful co-workers. There are also some notable differences. The war has become more real to her. She speaks of a patient who learns of having lost his fifth brother. She tells of having received, as gifts, a German ammunition wallet, a ribbon from a German Iron Cross medal, and various badges. It is her words, however, about a recent battle which stand out. Canadians have met the Germans in hand-to-hand combat in no man's land and "great was the slaughter of the enemy. Canada may well be proud of her sons." The lady from Centreville, New Brunswick, has neither any illusions nor any qualms about what is actually going on.

August 22, 1917
France

Dear All of You,

I must write you all though at times my inclination is to write to you separately for there are so many personal things to say yet it is stupid to repeat myself and there is so little to say. Today, three letters came—a long one from Uncle Charlie, one from Guy Fitz-Rudolph who is in Folkestone and a perfect one from mother written on July 30th. I cannot tell you how happy letters make me where there is a background of sadness and also all good things must be overshadowed for us temporarily. Why should we be excepted when all suffer, some so greatly. We have on Ward 5 an officer who has just heard of the death of his fifth brother. He did not tell me—it was a friend who visited him today, yet he always has a smile and an answer ready for me. Though he is always very quiet and is a journalist by profession and has a strong, fine face. and a Canadian—an exception, for most of our patients so far have been Englishmen or Scotchmen.

So far I have not since leaving home seen a death or a patient in critical condition. It is beautiful here and the sisters are friendly and attractive and most of the men, and there are many who are well worth knowing. Last night, after a very good concert given by seven men recovered from shell-shock, the CO brought a number of officers to the sisters mess for refreshments. There were few of us to entertain them but matron sent me off with great firmness to a certain corner to rescue a swarm of my officers from London. However, having no choice, they accepted the relief offer with perfect grace and presently I found myself the centre of a merry group. At our parting, they asked me to adopt them, which, of course, I accented.

I have been to a town not far from here where there is a small hospital, two sisters only (English) and the hospital is in a most wonderful old Chateau lent by a bankrupt duchess who lived there alone with her servants. A wonderful garden and old banqueting hall in ruins—15th century and a castle keep of the 11th century. The whole place is surrounded by wall and moat, with wonderful gate and towers, in one of which the sisters have their room and from a window in a deep stone wall look out upon a great dark forest in which are wild boars. Some of the patients are in the Chateau and others in a tent. I've been seeing visions ever since.

Another day we visited an aerodrome, saw aeroplanes ascend and descend, and later, as evening fell, saw flashes of shells bursting. Another day we rode some distance, had afternoon tea and badminton and returned to a concert given by a onetime patient. So you see we are a very happy family. When we want a little variety in the way of food, we walk to town, fifteen minutes from here and at the British Expeditionary Canteen get anything. We wish you could see the place. In the centre of numerous huts and vehicles a great tent with shelves and shelves of canned and bottled eatables, also biscuits, etc and books and drinks. No booze of course. I wish I could go into more detail but that will have to wait.

I'm afraid I've struck a permanent job as dietitian[19] for the officers wards. It is not easy and there is not a sister in the place who would exchange places with me. Matron Wilson is very kind and gives me all the assistance that she can, also the C.O. is very encouraging. By the way, he is Col. Reason, of London, Ont. I discovered today that Vernon Lamb (Capt) on the medical staff is here. I have not as yet seen him. He is a nephew of aunt Georgies, Marguerite's brother.

We are so very cosy in our tent. Tonight I heated water on the oil stove and had such a delightful sponge bath. You must never think of me as enduring hardships. I am enjoying a natural, wholesome life and such an interesting one. If I could only picture the whole thing for you.

Aeroplanes are no unusual sight hovering over our heads and sometimes doing very spectacular things for our benefit. Since the rain has ceased, our forces seem to be doing wonders along the front—everything is encouraging and this year there are not nearly so many casualties among our men. Two days ago they tell us our men went over the parapet somewhere beyond Vimy Ridge and met the Germans in a hand to hand fight in no man's land and great was the slaughter of the enemy. Canada may well be proud of her sons.

Dorothy is on night duty at present. I miss her much though the other sisters are so nice and worth cultivating. What a splendid time we shall have when this war is over. There has never been such joy in our lives as that will be. Yet you would not have me at home now I know. Send me any magazines you may have to spare. I mean like the Digest or Life or the Montreal Star once in awhile or the Telegraph, just something that will keep me in touch with the American continent and home.

I am so glad for Aunt Celia, Mary and Kathleen that they have had the boys home but I do hope this letter will find her in Centreville. Tell Alice to write Lee my address. I want to keep in touch with him. Send his to

19 The army had learned the importance of diet in the overall recovery of men exhausted and malnourished by life in the trenches. Pauline's position as dietician was a new one, but one which was critical to the restoration of the men.

me. My love to all my village friends. I think of them often and always when I write home. I hope by this time you have received the English photos. Tell Mildred to send me some gossip if she loves me and thank Florence for her letter. Heaps of love to all, Polly

I will find out about cabling money. It may be I can send what I have in England to Canada. I am spending very little, but mean to keep warm and well fed. There is no sign of famine here. From the wall of the citadel one looks on field after field of wheat and grain, cut, gathered and stacked—a bountiful harvest and very beautiful. I am seeing Millets and Corots in life—surely as lovely as the artist's conception which I hope one day to feast my eyes upon.

I have been given a German ammunition wallet and a bit of the ribbon that is always attached to the Iron Cross—also some badges. The ribbon is black and white corded silk. Now I must go to dreamland and you all know with whom that dear land is peopled. Heaps of love once more. By the way, Red Cross supplies are very much in evidence here so don't lose heart. The Red Cross Societies without doubt are doing their bit and helping to win the war and those who take no interest are missing the opportunity of a life time. Please see that I have Foster Scholey's, Fred Gibson's and George Long's address.[20] P'line

Congratulations to the trio of unfortunates who chose July 4th as a natal day. However, there are compensations no doubt, particularly for Sandy who I am delighted to learn has been appreciated by the many who have known his kindness in time of trouble. I hope Dr Peppers got my card from England.

P. B.

A note a few days later confirms that, although not her choice, Pauline is stuck with the dietician's job. She and Baldie apparently have less time

---

20 Foster B. Scholey (13787) and Fred Gibson (706777) were both born in Centreville, New Brunswick. Although Foster was living in Alberta and Fred in British Columbia, both had joined up and were doing their bit overseas.

off each day, and so are making the most of an hour or so by playing tennis—apparently despite the need to chase balls.

August 28, 1917
No. 3 Canadian Stationary Hospital, BEF, France

Dearest Mother and Dad,

Just a line tonight because always you are my last thought and my first on waking. I received my budget of letters today, including Jack's and one from Kathleen, also Mary's. It is more than good to hear—just heaven! I am not homesick, so much more contented to be doing something even if it must needs be very little.

I think I told you that I am at present Diet Nurse on the Officers Wards, not the part I would choose, but that which I have been appointed to do, I must do willingly, so I try to be content. We, Baldie and I, walk daily on our hour off or in the evening and are going in for tennis, so we are keeping in fine condition. This paper is exciting me to say things not becoming to a lady, upon it my pen almost refuses to make an impression.

There is little to tell. If I could speak of all the little things you would know there is much brightness in my days in spite of a rainy summer. The officers are adorable, mostly boys of twenty odd, some older, interesting, gay and brave. I have several nice souvenirs that I wish I might send. The best is a paper cutter made by a Lieutenant of the [Royal Flying Corps] from a bit of wire and screw of his machine. I told you, I think, of the bit of ribbon from an Iron Cross taken from a German by one of my patients.

The report from the lines are so encouraging. I think we all feel much cheered. Love to everybody. I will write again soon.

Daughter.

PAULINE D. BALLOCH

Pauline and Baldie continue to tramp about France in their heavy boots, exploring sights and buying supplies for the ward. The biggest news is of a trip to a nearby city (Albert) and seeing the famous cathedral and its leaning steeple-top statue. This scene was often photographed by official photographers and appeared on innumerable postcards. The superstition arose that if the statue ever fell, France would lose the war—French engineers and their cables made sure it stayed in place. What Pauline does not tell her parents, however, is that the trip took them twenty miles closer to the front. This was the reason the four Canadian nursing sisters were the only females in the French hotel's dining room, and the truth behind her statement to her parents that "[s]ome day we shall have great joy in talking this all over."

September 3, 1917
France

Dear Home People,

Just a line before turning in for the night. Things are pretty much as usual and life, in a way, very uneventful. However, yesterday we did get away for a few hours to a nearby city—about 20 miles and saw a famous cathedral, of which I have some pictures, and some day will send some cards. We also had a famous dinner, (famous in quite another sense), dining in a French hotel, filled with English officers, ourselves and two other Canadian sisters the only other feminine guests. We came home early, of course, in the moonlight, along a road bordered with fruit trees instead of poplars.

Tonight, Baldie and I, directly after supper, started off on a tramp, feet encased in heavy boots, a necessary part of our equipment, the roads are so hard, cobblestones and macadamized. We walked at a good swinging pace for about an hour and a quarter, besides which I walked to town today for supplies for the dining room of the Officers Ward, and endless running about the place—so you see I get plenty of exercise. I love all the letters I get though they don't come oftener than I like, still I get then fairly regularly and enjoy them more than I can ever say.

Last night we heard the guns for some time. It is not often that their roar reaches us. I wish you could see how cosy we are in our tents. Some day we shall have great joy in talking this all over and it is not so far away. Love to all, hope Aunt Celia will come to you later. I am glad Cassie Carr got to see you and is better. My love to Woodstock friends. I had a nice long letter from Aunt Cass. If I can ever find time I am going to write Elizabeth. The greatest deprivation we have here is no time by oneself for quiet thought. There is always someone with one.

Best love to Alice and Mildred and all my heart for my very own, including always sister Mary. Hope Guy will write me another interesting letter. I thoroughly enjoyed him on the Conscription question.

Lovingly Paul

Still living in a crammed tent, Pauline writes requesting supplies for the coming winter. She shares news that they will be housed under corrugated-iron-roofed huts once winter arrives. She mentions leaving her camera in England due to security concerns and a ban on their use on the continent. Her paragraph on the activity she sees daily in Doullens is an excellent description of what went on in a major transportation hub behind the lines. Her description of the British Empire at war in France is a perfect period piece of prose by a proud member of that Empire doing her bit.

September 8, 1917
France

Dear Dad,

Your letter of August 13 came today, so you see, it has been nearly four weeks on the way, not such a long time after all. I am so thankful you are getting my letters regularly and that the gloves and tie from London reached you and that mother likes her blouse. Also I sent a few trifles for Helen in your case and hope they have reached you. Someday I shall remember Guy and Mary, but it may be some time yet. I wrote a list of things I would be glad to have, warm socks for the winter and such, but don't think of sending anything else. We have no room for superfluities. Books or magazines at Christmas for we can't get too much to read, and perhaps a fruit cake, but other than these things for present needs, anything else is only an encumbrance. We have no place for storing extras. With the difference that I am living in a tent in France, I am living a normal life such as you would wish for me and there is positively no reason for any anxiety. I am as well off and as safe as in England and quite content.

I am grieved to learn of Mr Thistles' trouble. I will remember Mrs Thistles depression during the last weeks at home and his anxiety about the swelling in her throat. Although his sojourn in our town was so short she will be much missed and I wonder how poor Mr Thistle will bring up his delightful family of boys without her.[21]

It is good to hear about all home doings. I am so glad Jean is with you and will look forward to his letter. I know it will be a full one. It is said we will be in huts this winter, corrugated iron roofs, very comfortable and snug, but I hope we continue to live in tents til the end of October at least.

Last night we motored to a nearby village about 6 miles distant and

21 They were possibly Thomas and Annie Thistle, listed on the 1911 census as thirty-seven and thirty-four years of age, respectively, with four young boys: Claire, ten; John, six; Donald, two; and Eldon, ten months .

visited an old French Chateau, temporarily a hospital, a most interesting old place, fortified with gate and towers. It has an old eleventh century keep and banqueting hall, a wonderful garden, all a delight to one from a new country like ours.

We seldom hear the guns, but are quite accustomed to the whir of flying machines and motorcycles. All the activity we see is army activity, of course, great transport wagons and tenders, men tramping and on horseback, Australians, New Zealanders, Canadians, English, Scotch, Irish, Indians, with turbaned heads, les poilus in blues, countless soldiers of all descriptions, Chinamen at work on the roads and quite often, German prisoners.

I am going to mail you a post card now and again. Let me know if you get them. I feel quite sure they will be passed as they can furnish no information of use to the enemy supposing they should be intercepted. I have a few snaps taken in England but do not know if they will be allowed to go through and don't want to lose them. Will try one of myself someday. We are not allowed to use Kodaks here, and I gave mine up while here. It is just ten o'clock and the bugle has sounded "lights out." We have such a good bugler. It is lovely to be wakened in the morning by the sound of the "Reveille." You would love it too.

I am going very soon to send out a letter in search of Lee. I want to get in touch with him. His number and battery should find him anywhere. Will be glad to have any of the home boys addresses. A box of sweets or cakes from here would be sure to reach them and might cheer them considerably. Also they might be glad to know I am near even if I cannot see them. Has George Long come to France?

Guy Fitz-Randolph is in Folkestone and anxious to hear. I must write. Will write again in a few days even if I have little to say.

Heaps of Love, Pauline

Pauline might be but a nurse and not a general, but her appreciation of things military is expanding exponentially. She notes the dreadful effects of rain on the ability of troops to make progress. Her words would prove tragically prophetic as the "rule" changes on movement were a precursor to the Third Battle of Ypres, or Passchendaele. Her description of the weekly French "market" where she buys supplies for her ward and of the social life with doctors at the nearly chateau hospital are most vivid. Her reading of the bubbles in tea cups and her resultant popularity speak volumes about her ability to meet her co-workers' physiological needs. Who among present-day readers knows what in the world is a taradiddler?

September 13, 1917
No. 3 Canadian Stationary Hospital, BEF, France
Dear Home People,

September has brought us a delightful change in weather and we are basking in the warm rays of a cheery sun. Alas that sol was so persistently unfriendly during the month of August. The heavy and continuous rains make it very difficult for our brave men to accomplish the stupendous tasks set for them. This is perhaps the greatest discouragement of all and of course it will take days for the sun to undo the evil that has been wrought by the rain.

However, with us in the immediate vicinity, we lead almost as usual a life as at home, except that there are many restrictions. We get out for walks of course and have been permitted up to date to drive to nearby towns when the opportunity presented itself. However, it seems that is no longer to be allowed and we are all very sorry, though we can still find many pleasant things to do—one of which I shall proceed to tell you about so that you may see that we have jam with our bread and butter.

On Monday afternoon (just before the new rules were made) we were invited to picnic at a nearby hospital, about six miles away, the one I described to you some time ago; castle wall and fortified gates, eleventh century keep crumbling to ruins, but still standing grim and forbidding against a forest of green. An old banquet hall, only the ruins of the front remaining and the shell of an ancient church and tower. The officers play at badminton on a cinder court within so it has found a use once more.

We had a wonderful afternoon. Captain Manchester, our host, an M.D. from Vancouver and who knows Jack was very kind and interesting. He said Jack had taken him into the interior on a two week trip; that he had caught and broken a bucking bronco, the first to master the beast and he said a finer piece of riding he had never seen. We had tea on a grassy slope without the wall, looking down upon an orchard and, in the valley, the village beyond, numerous small patches of green and yellow—fields with a rich yield of various grains, and behind us the forest of enchantment in which lurked the wild boar. It was a lovely afternoon and our pleasure was not diminished by being an unusual one.

Today I went marketing. The French women bring their vegetables and eggs to the town square every Thursday and truly the things to be had today made one's mouth water. I was buying green stuff for the ward I am on—chicory (something like lettuce) melons, cucumbers, green leaves. It was great fun.

I hope you aren't worrying about me. We are so cosy and comfortable in our tent and later will be snug in huts. I am longing for something Canadian to read and if it is possible would like the Weekly Star, not the daily, it would only accumulate. Give my love to everybody. I often think of the village en masse, you may be sure you are never out of my thoughts.

This evening the staff officers are entertaining us, cards and dancing, does not sound like war does it? I usually do not go but am going in for it tonight. I hope you are as well and happy and contented as I, I could not wish you more. Tell Rhoda Sullivan that I have won a reputation as a fortune teller, that I once, on arriving, weakly yielded to a foolish wish that I read a cup and have since been progressing rapidly. I am becoming an outrageous taradiddler and can usually satisfy hunger for a bubble of this description. Yesterday a fairly sensible old girl saved her cup all afternoon for me to read and even the men (some of them only, thank goodness) seem to need a little teacup management. I am going to have conscientious scruples in future. It is dinner time and I must away. Love to Jean and Aunt Caroline.

Oceans of love to all, Pauline

The following is perhaps the most personally revealing letter of all. What does she feel, as a thirty-six-year-old single woman, surrounded by all these young men—men who were living a time of reprieve before returning to face death at the front yet again? She communicates her joy of dancing, while reflecting with wonder on her response to several ribald performances which saw her laugh "extravagantly." Certainly Pauline was no stranger to introspection! Finally, her remarks about her day spent with an adventurous young captain and about the grey hairs she sees in her mirror give us a glimpse of a lady not without regrets.

Friday Night, September 14, 1917
France

I had an unusually good time last night, one very good dance, two or three fairly good, but pleasant partners and three or four performances that should have been taboo. As usual, I found the latter amusing, (why I know not for they were neither graceful nor comfortable) and I laughed extravagantly. Today I had an afternoon at large and took care of an adorable youth, who is a captain and is now an instructor in a camp nearly after having done his bit (or part of it) at the line. We went tramping, bought peaches and ate them in the road and on the way home climbed down a steep bank to the river that would have tempted me in my teens, (in this adventurous one's company), if life still had (romantic) chances for me. I played the mountain goat to the life and felt quite a "kid"—still my mirror tonight insists that my hair is grey, not black. But what does it matter. We have had cocoa and biscuits in our tent entertaining the sisters in the neighbouring tents and now are ready for sleep. May your sleep be as sound as mine.

With love that bridges the Atlantic, devotedly, Pauline

Pauline writes of German prisoners building their winter huts and of a visit from an American baseball team. The Americans won. As to their attitude, she notes that they had not yet been to war and suffered and died and sacrificed on the massive scale that the British Empire and the French had done. She notes dryly, however, that, although they needed lots of encouragement to join the struggle, she is sure they will make a significant difference. Pauline's comments on light casualties at the time are odd, but the rain and resultant agony of the Passchendaele struggle would soon change her tone.

October 4, 1917
France

Dear Mother and Father,

I have been sending cards this week, a booklet of postals and two other cards and hope they have found you. There is so little to say really and yet I know you cannot hear often enough, nor at great enough length.

Our huts are being put up by German prisoners and will soon be ready for us and so we shall be snug and warm for the winter. However, we are not yet tired of our tents and you would be astonished to see how comfortable we are.

Yesterday we were visited by a large number of Americans. The U.S. Army Medical Corps baseball team played against the CAMC here. The game was watched with great interest and enthusiasm by all, including patients who were able to be out. Some were carried out in their beds that they might look on at the game and it is splendid that their minds could in such fashion be got away from the war and its consequences. You can scarcely understand how away from the war we really seem to be, though said to be "in the field"—a very broad term by the way.

The game was played at the base of the rampart in an enclosure formed by an irregularity in the wall, the outline of which is like a star. We, the onlookers, were high up on the point, a triangular lawn, the two sides of which are outlined by fine trees and from the base or third side of which triangle we looked down upon the game. The U.S. won by a score of 9 to 5—encouraging for them and they don't quite need encouragement—tho' they did need coaxing to get them into the war. Now in it, they make all the difference in the world.

Isn't it good to watch the German line gradually being pushed back? We are surely winning, if slowly and suffering fewer losses also and our gains in Mesopotamia and Africa are encouraging as well. Truly it cannot go on much longer and I feel sure next Spring will find the victory admittedly ours. Watch out for a little souvenir for Dad's birthday. It will be only a trifle.

I wish I had more photographs, there are many I would like to remember, but am afraid I can't afford it just now. I dare say Henry Lee and Rhoda and Margaret Adams and Rigby and one or two others would like one as a souvenir, but it will have to be later, if at all. Meanwhile here are one or two snaps taken in Orpington. Do you like them? Now I must to sleep. Does it give you comfort to know I am diet sister? It isn't half as nice as nursing.

Daughter Jane

Not having heard from home for two weeks, Pauline rejoices at having received mail, but has to correct her parents' impression of the danger she is in. She assures them again of her safety and that the Allies are winning the war. She comments on the cost of food, including eggs, and, as thoughts of upcoming Christmas parcels begin to percolate, asks for little from home. Perhaps as an extra consolation to her parents, she mentions the visit of the Anglican bishop of New Westminster, British Columbia, and the words of encouragement he had for the boys. Finally, she mentions sending back through the hospital system four very ill patients who would be returned to England. She adds that three of the men were very young—in their early twenties—but she had grown to adore them, although she adds sadly that she most likely will never see them again.

October, 8, 1917
France

Dear Ones,

A long letter yesterday from mother after a silence of nearly a fortnight to gladden my heart. The activity along the front has had its effect upon the mail which has not been coming quite so regularly so we are all looking forward to a tardy budget. The postal card referred to is of one of the roads leaving this town and the trees are Lombardy poplars. I sent it because it is typical of the roads here. This is not the loveliest part of France yet we see many beautiful things. I have sent also a book of views and a few other postals. I also have enclosed one or two snaps taken in England which I trust have reached you.

I only wish I might send you more detailed accounts of everything. One thing your letter proves to me—the wrong idea you have of my condition from reading the papers. You speak of the "slight hold" I have, yet I am more safe here than in England, as safe, perhaps, as at home. The line is continually advancing, leaving us daily a little farther behind. The bombs we hear are from a nearby trench mortar school. Only a few times have we heard the explosions from the line. The most exciting sounds we hear come from the aeroplanes that fly above us daily. Two nights ago eighteen lads stopped over because of bad weather and came to our mess for a little fun.

We expect to be here for the winter and so you may rest happy in our security. Keep well for my sake and it won't be so very long before we shall be having a jolly reunion. There is no doubt that we are winning the war.

The letter you enclosed is the first of a series of four written by an Australian boy in an effort to hear from me. His last one found me and of course I wrote him. He had been in the trenches since 1914 when he got his "Blighty" which brought him to Orpington.

You ask me what to send—a fruit cake and nice box of Mildred's fudge, also a box of Cliff's roasted peanuts, as dad suggests, and books at any time. Nothing else that I can think of.

I know things are very high. Prices here are awful, eggs; 6 are 7 cents apiece, (30 to 35 centimes). I am sorry Jean is so miserable. Indeed she has not been well for a long time and has had much to rob her of her health. Dear Aunt Caroline had made great sacrifices but she has this to console her; Wilmot and myself will be comparatively safe. I wrote Uncle Charlie a few days ago. It is comforting to know he is not far away. You must give my love to all my village friends. I often think of them.

We have just sent some lads on to the base hospital and from there they will get to England for they have been very ill. One is a man of thirty odd years, but the other three are boys who began in the ranks and won their commissions. One has been "over the top" nineteen times, seven times in divisional attacks, the remainder battalion, and never a scratch, but he came down with trench fever and has been ill for weeks. Now he will get home for leave and then back again.

I adore the three of them and they know it, tho' I shall perhaps never see them again. Usually the men, whether in the ranks or officers, are in their early twenties or younger.

Now it is time for me to turn in, but not until I tell you of our visit from the Bishop of New Westminster. He is at Etaples and came here to confirm a large class. He gave us a wonderful address—it must have helped the many men who heard him, besides he knew whereof he spoke for he has two sons in France. I think his name is Adam De Pencier. Mr Rigby will know.

Now good night and oceans of love, daughter

The following letter is an exception in that Pauline writes not to her parents, but to her sister-in-law Mary, her brother Guy's wife. She relates her opportunity to learn French, her thirst for expressly Canadian news, and her desire to taste a homemade, well-iced cake. Her mention of a trip to Amiens must be a separate excursion from the one she wrote about to her parents on September 3, for in that instance she was surrounded by British officers. Ironically, despite often hearing the term, Pauline was wrong to assume that napoo *was French slang— it is actually of Hindustani origin, just like the term "chit." Many of the regular British battalions had seen service in India before the war, where they had picked up convenient local slang and brought it with them to the fields of France and Flanders. What was meant is that Guy's camera was* kaput *or irreparably broken and useless.*

October 19, 1917
No. 3 Canadian Stationary Hospital, France

Dear Mary,

Just received your letter today with enclosed and with you agree that Guy's Kodak is "napoo," French slang, I believe for no good and I think should be considered not worthy such subjects as yourself and me. However the one of you upon the bench is worth having even if it does not do you justice—the "pose" is so pretty and natural, but the others are unspeakably awful.

Many thanks for sending them however. It is good to get things from home—home! How much it means and what visions the word breeds. So often my thoughts are with you and your anxiety for your mother and I wish I might do something to help and comfort. Alas, how limited we are. Please give her my love. When you write, tell her I think of her often.

We are not busy at present and may not be for some time as the fighting is farther north. It seems a pity to be here and not to be nursing with all ones might and nerve, but if it means fewer casualties we should be thankful. Someday if you want to please me send me a cake in a tin box with a nice thick icing. Several of the sisters have received cake from home and they were the most joyfully received of anything that has come. I am looking forward to receiving a Ladies Home Journal from home some day and a paper with some <u>Canadian</u> news.

We sometimes see the American officers. They are stationed about 16 miles from here. Four of us had lunch in Amiens not long ago and the room was full of Americans. I have begun to study French. Goodness knows how far I shall get with it but I have been fortunate in finding opportunity if I have the zeal to apply myself.

The Belgian priest who is here and one day found me with a French grammar got me to read a few sentences and insisted that I read as though I knew French. Of course, I thought it a joke and could hardly think him serious but he proved his sincerity by sending me to a French woman of breeding Madam de Reguelie who reads and writes English but cannot speak it and who wishes to exchange with me. I go to her tomorrow for tea and am to meet a friend who knows English well. Madame is a countess but has dropped her title. She is middle-aged and charming and has a daughter Suzanne of about sixteen or seventeen years. They live in a house not far from the citadel with a great garden at the back enclosed in the usual way by a high stone wall. She spends only two weeks out of each month in the town, the remaining two weeks with her husband who is in the French army. She is introducing me to her friend so she may help me in her absence. Are they not kind? It is to be hoped I shall profit by such a rare opportunity.

I am hoping each mail will bring me news of home. Do tell me of Guy and yourself. Your letters are such a treat. Now I must turn in. Tomorrow I shall write home but won't repeat this news as I know my letters are sent on.

Heaps of love, Pauline

The next day Pauline writes her parents. Things are quiet for the moment and while her assumptions concerning casualties, especially up north in Flanders, will prove tragically wrong, for the moment, she has spare time. She tells of the circumstances surrounding her opportunity to learn French and confesses she starts from a point where she "knows nothing of the language."

October 20, 1917
France

Dear Mother and Father,

A letter was written and sent by me to Mary yesterday and it is surely your turn today. Indeed there is plenty of time for writing as we have few patients, comparatively, at present. Indeed, report has it that such is the case universally. However, I am busy in a way that will surprise you and please you too. It seemed too bad to have spare time and not utilize it so I grasped an opportunity that came to be in quite a surprising way. Not long ago, I was relieving for a night sister for a couple of hours in the evening and because there was little to do took with me a

French grammar that I found here in one of the shops. While I was busily engaged making its acquaintance in comes the French padre, or rather he is Belgian, and he showed much interest in my effort. He insisted that I read for him and then assured me that I was making an unusually good attempt at the pronunciation and thought me much farther advanced than I am. As you know, I know nothing of the language. However, he proved his sincerity. Some days later a French woman of refinement with her daughter called on me with the result that I have visited their house and am to go there as often as possible for our mutual advantage. They read and write English but cannot speak well. Our first meeting was "tres difficile" and we had to extricate ourselves from a series of dilemmas by writing much and often. Next time I took afternoon tea with them and met a friend of theirs who speaks English very well. Madame de Reguelie and her daughter go away on Tuesday to spend a fortnight with Madame's husband who is a French officer and this friend insists that I go to her as often as possible for lessons. They are so kind and interested that I think I must surely be able to learn something and what I do learn will be Parisian.

Today I walked with Mademoiselle Suzanne de Reguelie and we exchanged limited remarks on the beauty of the sky and country, on cows and horses and railroads and such things of great interest. I am translating each day a few lines of Breves nouvelles d'aujourd'hui and find myself each day the richer by two or three words and as the saying goes—every little bit helps.

I hope you are not anxious about me. There's no occasion as you would know if you were here. I haven't heard from Lee—perhaps he did not get my letter. Where does Alice send his letters? I also wrote Keith MacGowan[22] and hope he will receive my note.

22 Keith C. MacGowan, born 1890, Charlottetown, Prince Edward Island, joined the 131st Battalion in New Westminster, British Columbia, in May 1916, transferred to the 47th Battalion, became a captain, and was awarded the Military Cross at Vimy Ridge; before war's end, he added two bars to the medal, one for Passchendaele and another for Valenciennes.

The sisters are such pleasant girls and I am becoming much attached to some of them. Dorothy has just come off night duty. I am so glad to have her again, she is such a cheery soul. Miss River, who is in charge of the Officers Ward at present is a dear and very interesting. She is Scotch, red hair, a clergyman's daughter and brimming with character. Miss White is her friend, she is English, but both have lived a few years in Canada. I hope you are keeping warm and well. Do take care of yourselves. I am terrified when I think of the mad youthful things you so often indulge in. I am sending a card once in a while. Hope they reach you.

Heaps of love Daughter

Pauline's big news is that they have moved into their winter quarters: Nissen huts. Better than tents, but far from palatial, she describes in minute detail the interior decorating she has performed on her room number six. In answer to her parents' questions, she attempts to describe her work which, to her regret, is not direct nursing. She is continuing her French lessons, but the stark reality of the war again intrudes: her temporary instructor is a lady who has lost both her lands and her husband to the Germans. The hospital continues to send troops away, this time not to England. but back to the front to fight yet again.

October 26, 1917
France

Dear Father and Mother,

Often as I write to you I suppose my letters are not frequent enough and perhaps once in awhile one goes astray or is a long time finding you. Yet I think, considering the times, mail is very satisfactorily carried.

We moved into our huts on the 24th—such comfort. Our hut is very long with a corridor about 4 ft wide all along the front and entered by three doors. The rooms, ten in number, open off the corridor. Mine is number 6 with a wide, shallow window about 5 ft from the floor from which I look over the rampart at miles of rolling country, farms and woodland and in the distance, an aerodrome. Nissen huts, that may be incorrectly spelt.

My room is about 12 ft sq I should think, painted a deep rose hew. I have a very comfortable bed, with plenty of bedding, a warm blanket on the floor, a dressing table made of packing boxes, a washstand (ditto), a folding camp chair and a trunk disguised with my rug as a very comfy sitter (set-two), a brand new Red Cross Oil stove that warms me in a flash and heats water for my bird bath. As well, a green lantern with a candle, window curtains of cheese cloth and drapery of black and white, blue and heliotrope design, cretonne. I am expecting some old rose fabric with which I shall make a wardrobe and improvise a chair and cosy corner out of more packing boxes. On my walls are some pictures cut from magazines, two maps of our battle front, a sketch or two and my two dearest at my head just where I can see them before going to sleep. I could not be more comfortable, nor better and am oh so grateful for the privilege of being here.

You ask just what my work is. That is not easy to tell. I wish it were nursing, but it is making the menu for the day, buying a few extras, such as fresh eggs, fresh fish, vegetables and fruit that cannot be supplied by the quartermaster's department. Seeing that things are probably cooked and served and providing diet for sick patients. You ask if it is likely to be a permanent post. One can never tell. Most fervently I trust not. The chances are all against any change for me this autumn and perhaps this winter. So rest happy. We have been sending away many patients of late—such dear boys. This morning three went up the line to do their bit in the thick of it once more. Most of the men who come in here go back to fight again. Splendid fellows! You know what a privilege it is just to be here and help a little when one may!

The gains to the north and by the French in the south have been so magnificent and so encouraging. We are most surely winning. We sometimes see American officers—engineers. They have yet to make the sacrifice that is an old story with Great Britain and France.

My friend Madame de Regueliu and Suzanne have gone to Abbeville for a fortnight—a friend of theirs, Madame de Leoncour asked me for tea today. They are so very anxious to help me with French. Madame de Leoncour has been widowed by this cruel war. She came here from Lens with her two small children, "Jacques et Jean"—left all her property in the hands of Germans and her husband dead. She is cheerful and sweet. Wonderful! She speaks a pretty English, very correct, but with a decidedly French accent. She loves to read English books. I am to visit her again on Monday. Le pere Perot, who sent me to them has returned from his leave.

Now I must get to sleep. May your sleep be as sound as mine and as dreamless.

Your loving daughter

Again Pauline finds herself reassuring her parents of her well-being, then switches topic. As for religion, Pauline, who is Church of England (Anglican), tells her parents that her unit is losing its beloved chaplain, Major John Cheyene Davidson, who was worn out and had been called home by his bishop. The fifty-seven-year-old chaplain had joined up in March 1916, but neither he nor his bishop envisioned the war's lasting so long or being so brutal. Although his parish had declined in his absence and his bishop was clamouring for his return, he was still loath to go. He knew the greater need was in the hospital wards of France, among the wounded men and the valiantly struggling staff.

Nov., 3, 1917
France

Dear Father and Mother,

I must write at once to thank you for the woollen things, they will be such a comfort to me this winter. You will be glad to know that I wear warm stockings and heavy boots. I have had my stout walking boots resoled and am now quite accustomed to their weight. At first, they seemed very clumsy but without doubt they are a very great protection. We walk long distances sometimes, at least home people would think them long, but the exercise is good for us and the fresh air keeps us fit. It was very kind of the ladies to knit for me and I shall write each one. The stockings fit well and are very comfortable.

I wish you might see our hut now that we are settled. Our rooms look cosy and are very warm. I sent to England for old rose satin and my furniture made of boxes with chintz covering and hangings of old rose, makes a very comfy looking room.

This life agrees with me. So that as far as I am concerned you have nothing to be anxious about. It seems to me I am always writing about myself, trying to reassure you, but I don't want you to worry when there is no occasion.

I have heard from Guy and Mary and know of their going south. I think it is a very wise move, but my heart goes out to dear Mary. I know how sad her heart has been because of her mother's long and hopeless illness and even as I write they may have come to the parting. I cannot be thankful enough for the years of comparative health and great happiness that have been given us.

We are letting our dear old Padre, Major Davidson go back to his home in Peterborough, Ontario. They are sending for him as his church has suffered so in his absence, but he is very loath to go even so, for he thinks the greatest need is here. However, his health is such that it is advisable that he go back. He is not young and has such tremendous energy, that he does not spare himself and consequently has overworked. We all love him and think him a saint.

That reminds me, there is a wonderful book, a great favourite of his, that you must get and read. It would be a delightful and worthwhile Christmas gift for Mary or Guy or Helen—"The Student in Arms" by Donald Hankey.

Major Davidson has a sister in Toronto married to Mrs George Hanning's brother. Of course, he knows my Toronto friends well. He was born in Prince William. He is second cousin of Canon Elligood in Montreal and knows all the old Fredericton names.

We, five of us sisters, most from Scotland, Miss White, English, Miss Jukes, Vancouver, Dorothy and myself, dined him at Gezaincourt two nights ago—we had delicious soup, omelette, chicken, potatoes, soufflé and pears. It was great fun and our delightful guest was at his best, described his reception in England (Margate) in a way that should have been taken in shorthand, so perfect and amusing was the whole thing. I would like to try and write it down someday only I can never do justice to the humour. He has asked the sisters who are off duty to have tea with him on Monday. I hope I shall be free.

My friend Madame de Regueliu returns on Wednesday. Don't fancy me making any great progress. I am a great blockhead since leaving school but may understand something of the language by the end of the winter. Now I must to work again. We are not very busy, but are needed just the same, they tell me so I try to be content. My love to all my dear friends in Centreville. I hope they come to you sometimes to gossip about me.

Heaps of love, Pauline

As the Battle of Passchendaele rages on to the north in Flanders, Pauline pens a short but telling note. One of her colleagues, Miss Muir, has returned from a shift only to find a notice of her brother's death during the latest Canadian advance. Another nursing sister has lost four out of seven brothers. Not surprisingly Pauline tells her parents that she retreated to the quiet of her room, and there alone spent two hours of seclusion rereading letters from her beloved parents. This gave her some comfort and solace while surrounded by so much tragedy and sorrow.

November 8, 1917
No. 3 Canadian Stationary Hospital, BEF, France

Dear Father and Mother,

I have had the afternoon off duty, so after having a French lesson with Mademoiselle Rawstone, I looked over my old home letters and with you spent quite two delightful hours. Your letters do me so much good, they are so worthwhile, expressive of your dear selves. I am longing for the time to come when I am to return and coddle you but we must be patient for there is so much to be done first and you would not recall me now. I often think of Mary and the sorrow that is her portion now.

I am very fond of the sisters I am working with, particularly Miss Muir of whom I have spoken before. Poor girl, a tragic message awaited her when she came off duty today—one of her brothers had been killed in the latest Canadian advance. She has two others in active service. Another sister, out of seven brothers in Khaki, has lost four. She is a marvel of pluck and good cheer. This old world is mother of many fine children. Baldie hasn't heard from her brother for weeks. She is pretty anxious at times though she says nothing. I trust she will be spared bad news.

We have had a lovely letter from our 'English Mother'—so Miss Robinson signs herself, with a snap of herself enclosed for me, holding in her arms Mrs Bliss's baby (Mrs Bliss is her sister)—I want to keep it yet I would like to send it to you that you may see how sweet she is, so someday you may find it in a letter.

Now good-night and heaps of love, daughter

Apparently, Pauline had received a letter from her mother wherein her spelling was corrected—she loves this particular motherly touch. On a more serious note, she mentions all the severe fighting that is going on—by the boys and, in some instances "mere infants," to use her terminology. Pauline, however, is not naïve—these men are fighting both their Empire's battles and the temptations of the world. The last thought brings her to the topic of the bishop of Fredericton's tour. Bishop Richardson is in England on behalf of all Canadian Anglican bishops, and will also come to France to speak to the boys. Whether the troops found his words as comforting as Pauline hopes, is at best, doubtful. Many men assessed the home front clergy's uninformed enthusiasm as somewhere between totally out of touch and outright repugnant. Chaplains who actually saw the front and those who shared in the troops' deprivations and dangers fared far better in the soldiers' estimation both at the time and in the post-war years.

November 1917

Dear Mother,

I have read and re-read your letter many times. It is so full of everything I wanted to hear and your writing is so clear and beautiful. I like to be told about the misspelt (mich-spelt—no !!) words, but I do write in a great hurry and expect you will have much to over look along that line.

Dear Aunt Cass! It is a comfort to me to know that you three are together and I think that she is a brick to let Wilmot come. However, there is only one place for the young and physically fit and it is somewhere this side of the water. I hope someday to hear from Lee. I have heard twice from Keith and also from Noel. Don't fear about the latter. His wife is in England and I have no intention of flirting with him. Too bad he can't see me now with my hair in a psyche; spectacles and pyjamas, instant cure, guaranteed. If the worst comes to the worst, he shall have radical treatment, count on me. He's in the thick of it now, poor boy, and I hope will come out all right. At least we gain on the western front. For days the guns have been pounding, we can hear them for miles, and troops—cavalry, artillery, transports streaming through. Many changes in hospital which I cannot tell of, we shall soon have no patients left, and eighteen of our sisters go to casualty clearings tomorrow. I am one of the twenty-four left safe and comfortable within the walls of the citadel. Talk of being warm, a red-cross hot water bag warms my bed, Red Cross (RC) stockings, (bed socks) keep my tootsies comfy, a Red Cross oil stove heats my room. My furniture is made of RC boxes and an RC table holds my books and an RC chair my clothes.

As for the wards, it's RC equipment pretty nearly from start to finish. What our hospitals would do without the Red Cross, I fail to know. Their work is magnificent and indispensible to the hospitals. I think you do splendidly at home. Personally, I am most grateful for my stockings and they are being worn already. Be sure I shall take great care of them.

I have just had tea with some of the sisters; Baldie, Macdongall and Rose. I will finish this card and then to bed.

Do you hear from me often? You should hear at least twice a week, sometimes more frequently. I hope I shall see Bishop Richardson if he comes to France. If the boys fighting for their country are cared for and nurtured—the Church at home will prosper even if neglected for the present. The great need is here, poor boys, some are mere infants, and fighting our battles, plus the world's temptations.

My love to Centreville. It's on my heart with you and dad in the centre. Watch out for a bit of embroidery hand work and a letter opener for dad.

Shortly after the above letter, Pauline penned a short note to her mom. Her letter-writing time had been spent sending a note of thanks to the local Red Cross. In her estimation that organization was doing essential war-related work and making a notable contribution.

November 22, 1917
France

Dear Mother,

I have spent my time for letter writing today addressing Christmas cards and writing the enclosed to the Red Cross at home—so you and dad must wait a day or two for your letter. However, if my last had a fair crossing it should have reached you just two days in advance of this French message to Aunt Cass. Hope you get my box o.k. Love to everybody, P'line

I did promise A. Cody a photograph. If you have one to spare let her have it, if not, tell her I will remember her next time.

Paul

Mere days before Christmas 1917, Pauline writes her parents. White snow has temporarily covered the grey mud which surrounds them, and Christmas music livens the atmosphere, but it will be a difficult Christmas for thousands. All the nurses who had been called away to work at casualty clearing (advanced aid) stations dealing with the thousands of wounded from the Passchendaele battle will have returned by Christmas.

For the Past—
Remembrances.

For the Present—
Best Wishes.

For the Future—
Good Fortune.

From Ray McLeish
No. 3 Canadian Stationary Hospital

Matron	E. M. Wilson,	C.A.M.C.,	R.R.C.
N. Sister	L. Bell	C.A.M.C.,	R.R.C.
"	E. M. Best	"	
"	M. S. D. Beatty	"	
"	D. M. Y. Baldwin	"	
"	P. D. Ballock	"	
"	M. Bishop	"	
"	E. V. Cameron	"	
"	S. B. Cameron	"	
"	C. Cameron	"	R.R.C
"	C. E. Chisholm	"	
"	M. Chapman	"	
"	A. E. Donnelly	"	
"	K. F. Durkin	"	
"	M. S. Ellis	"	R.R.C.
"	K. Guerin	"	
"	K. E. Gray	"	
"	M. E. Hazard	"	
"	H. C. Jukes	"	
"	C. M. Latimer	"	
"	M. B. McElhoes	"	
"	B. O. Maguire	"	
"	M. E. McKenzie	"	
"	I. B. Muir	"	
	A. McDougall	"	
"	A. T. McLeod	"	
"	J. A. McDonald	"	
"	C. M. McKenzie	"	
"	M. M. Moore	"	
"	B. McDougall	"	
"	R. McLeish	"	
"	C. M. McLean	"	
"	H. A. McLaughlin	"	R.R.C.
"	F. D. McLaughlin	"	
"	H. V. Petrie	"	
"	E. L. Pringle	"	
"	P. Rose	"	R.R.C.
"	C. H. Ross	"	
"	E. M. Seely	"	
"	J. I. Smith	"	
"	E. V. Strange	"	
"	A. Sutherland	"	
"	L. C. White	"	
"	E. M. Young	"	
Home Sister	H. R. Michie	"	

Christmas
1917.

The Commanding Officer, Officers,
Nursing Sisters, Non-Commissioned Officers,
and Men
Unite in extending to you
Christmas Greetings & Best Wishes
for a
Glad New Year.

No. 3 Canadian Stationary Hospital,
B. E. F., France.

Inside of 1917 Christmas card for # 3 Canadian Stationary Hospital in France. Note the list of all the nursing staff, including Pauline and her friend NS Baldwin.

Pauline's Anglican connections continue to produce interesting encounters. Lieutenant John B. Wilkinson, the son of the minister at Springhill, New Brunswick (now part of Fredericton), is in the area and spending time with Pauline. Here, too, tragedy intrudes, for young Wilkinson has lost both a chum and a brother to the Passchendaele mud in the past month.

December 17, 1917
No. 3 Canadian Stationary Hospital BEF, France

Dear Dad and Mother,

A little more than a week and Christmas will be here. Never have we been so far away from each other at this time, but there are thousands of others in the same case with far less to comfort them. For you I believe are snug, comfortable and well and I am in such excellent condition that you should feel no anxiety concerning me. We are having our first snow. We have had frost of course though the ground has been frozen only on the surface, but today everything is white and lovely for the time being, a borrowed beauty that will vanish with the first warmth from the sun.

Things are pretty much with us as they have been with not much that one can write about. The sisters who have been to hospitals in need of reinforcements have nearly all returned, so we shall be all together for Christmas.

Two (Canadian) engineering Battalions have been in rest nearby one of the officers is Wilkinson—"Willie" Wilkinson's son.[23] He is such a nice chap, and seems to regard me as a sort of relation. We spent yesterday afternoon together and he is coming tonight for a band concert given by the 61st Div band. We are having such music these days—xmas time, it is lovely for us all, but splendid for our convalescent men. I wish I were on the nursing ward for xmas, however there is no hope, so I must try to content myself. Young Wilkinson has lost a brother, a cousin, and his chum since November. I must write Margaret.[24] I quite often see Captain Manchester and I like him very much. I have not heard from Ruth for some time. I am sending her a little xmas box which I hope will reach her.

Heaps of love, daughter Jane

23 John Bacon Wilkinson, born 1889, lieutenant in the 72nd Battery, CEF. His father was the Anglican minister at St. Peter's, Springhill, New Brunswick, at the time. His brother Lawrence Tremaine Wilkinson (335906), born 1893, died of his wounds near Ypres on October 30, 1917.
24 Margaret was a sister of the Wilkinson boys, born in 1884, so closer in age to Pauline.

Just before Christmas, Pauline writes her dad again. Her thoughts are more religious, with talk of a picture of Christ next to one of her parents and her thankfulness that Wilmot, Uncle Charlie and Aunt Caroline's son, was not in Halifax for the dreadful explosion but had sailed from there shortly before the disaster on December 6, 1917. On a considerably lighter note, she writes of all the goodies that are arriving in time for the celebration of Christmas.

December 18, 1917
France

Dear Dad,

I wrote so hurriedly my last letter that perhaps I did not mention that I have received two boxes from home—one with a cake which we have not yet sampled and such delicacies, cookies and socks; another with chocolates and books from mother, also warm mittens and the candles and candle sticks from you. In mother's letter she thinks you have received all my letters, that no week goes by without word from me. I am very glad but think a few must go astray as I write even more often than that, and shall continue to do so, hoping that no week shall pass without word from me.

I burn two nice candles nightly on either side of a picture of Christ given to me by Major Davidson before he left. They are on a mantle just opposite my bed and just above my head where I can see you as I go to sleep in a picture of yourself and mother. So I am constantly (visually) reminded of you, though that is not necessary as you know.

Thank Mildred and Aunt Cass for their share in the boxes. I have not made inroads on the sweets yet, but there's a sweet time coming. I remember you asked about my evening dress. I put it away somewhere when I went to Toronto. I have no idea where. I took only my black evening gown and cloak with me there and think they must still be in my hat box. The green neck must be in one of the other trunks. I certainly did not give it away. However, it does not matter much as it will be quite out of date before I can wear it again. I wish I were going to dress for dinner at home this year. However, it is pleasant to think of you as having Alice and Aunt Caroline on xmas day. By the time this reaches you aunt C's anxiety about Wilmot[25] will be over. If he is to be in Boulogne (Bouloin seems to be the popular pronunciation, though I have not yet asked Madame de Regueliu and may not see her until after xmas), I will make inquiries, but it is popularly as you wrote it, not as we thought it to be. I was relieved to hear that he was on the high seas and not in Halifax. Such a shocking disaster! I am awfully sorry to learn of Mr Rigby's accident and will write him today if possible, no doubt, by this time Helen is with him.

Now I must get on with my work, the same thing. I have had a lovely book from Mrs Fred Robinson, England, written from Ethelinda, Wales. Also cake and sweets from Mary, handkerchiefs from a Toronto aunt of Dorothy's—so you see xmas is already on its way. Heaps of love and Christmas wishes from Polly

I am spending very little, comparatively, and for yours truly, possibly because we are allowed only a limited amount, P'line

1918

Pauline's next letter, almost a month later, continues to speak of parcels received and of an apparent mix-up among the gifts she sent to Canada for Christmas, her father really not needing an embroidered corset! She has, however, two significant news items. First, she has finally been transferred off the Officers' Ward, and for this she is most thankful. Second, she and Baldie have dates for their much-anticipated leave to southern France later in January.

25 Wilmot B. Main (2605810), born in Edmundston, New Brunswick, 1890, and living in St. Stephen when he joined the CAMC in August 1917.

January 13, 1918
France

Dear Mother and Father,

Although you seem to think you get all my letters, "I haae me dooots" for I certainly write more than once a week and never let a fortnight go by without writing. So I shall try to send brief word at least twice or three times a week.

Mother's came yesterday telling me of the arrival of my little gift for you dad, with an embroidered corset cover. It, the latter, was meant for Mary and I cannot think how I failed to put her name on the wrapper. Evidently the letter explaining why I sent it to you has failed to reach you. I wanted you to see what beautiful work the French women do. I sent mother an embroidered linen scarf for the sideboard and hope by now you have it.

Our leave (Baldies and mine), is in for the 21st of Jan. We hope to spend it in Nice with Uncle Charlie. However, he may not get away when we do because of Wilmot's arrival and of course there is a doubt about our leave coming on time. However, I think you can be fairly sure of thinking of us as being in Nice at the ideal time of the year, drinking in the beauty of the blue Mediterranean and the southern flowers and perhaps seeing Monaco and Cannes, both not far from that lovely city. My only sorrow is that I am so far from you and that is not heavy so long as you keep well.

You may bank on my good health, I have never been better, and am not overworked and have plenty to eat of nourishing food. Christmas was a strenuous time, not because of strenuous nursing but because of xmas cheer. However, as I have told you, the patients had such a wonderful time and so we were all many times repaid.

I have received several boxes; one from Caroline Carr and one from Rachel, also the three from home, one from Mary, another from Ethelrude Oates, Ladies Home Journal from Ethelrude also and the xmas number from dad. I have just been taken from the Officers ward where I have been ever since my arrival—a long time and beginning to be very tiresome. I am glad of the change. You may think of me as having even lighter duty. When heavy duty comes I shall be quite ready for it and physically fit and shall be sure of my rest after. So do not ever waste your strength worrying about me. It is good to think of you as having aunt Caroline with you and I think a comfort to you all as well.

Today is like a spring day, very little snow, green moss on roofs and tree trunks, sun shining and warm. I will write again soon with your letters before me. Meanwhile all my love to you.

Daughter Jane

Although it is now February, Pauline has not as yet been on leave to the south of France. Uncle Charlie will not be joining them, for he was still waiting for his son Wilmot to arrive in France. Pauline is not just off the Officers' Ward; she is doing her turn of the dreaded "night duty," a responsibility which would last for a full month. Nonetheless, she is clearly content. Her time is passing pleasantly enough with the promise of both spring flowers and bicycle rides to come, and leave to the south of France preceding the advent of spring. There are no foreseen clouds on her horizon.

February 2, 1918
No. 3 Stationary Hospital, BEF, France

Dear Father and Mother,

I am wondering if you received my letter telling of the warm sunny days that we enjoyed during the last few days of January. Alas they were all too short and now we have instead heavy mist and the thermometer just low enough to frost the tress and walls, chilly weather, but it might be worse. I am thankful for warm clothing and under my apron am wearing the sleeveless sweater Mary sent me, and over all my blue sweater that I brought with me.

Another change has come to me and I am now on night duty—not too difficult and it will be for only one month, that is always the term of night duty here so one does not become tired out. Our leave for the south of France will not come through for another month. I am glad to get night duty over before going away. If we go to the south we shall be looked after all the way and will have to stay in a house for nurses while in Cannes. It won't be as free a time away but you can think of us as carefully guarded. It is a state of affairs I am not very keen about in my independent thirties. However, it will be restful and the Mediterranean in March is something to dream about. Don't think of me as making rapid progress in French. It will be months before I have even the rudiments, for of late, I have had little chance to see my friends and never hear it spoken. So as you can see it will be long before I could speak myself, but I am hoping to be able to read it quite easily by summer and to understand simple conversation even if I cannot join in.

It is disappointing that uncle Charlie could not get leave with us but I can well understand his wish to be in Boulogne when Wilmot arrives. Aunt Caroline must have rejoiced when she knew he had safely landed. The tragic occurrence at Halifax must have tried everybody at home, even those who had no friends there, and a shock such as it must have been, must have made an easy mind with Wilmot on the high seas, a difficult achievement for Aunt Caroline. However, I know what wonders she can accomplish in that time. One of my chief delights is picturing the three of you grouped about a cosy fire snug and well and as happy as may be in these days of cares, and somehow I think you are all happier than if you had the three of us at home fretting because we were not here.

In a few weeks this place is going to be delightful, it is always a romantic, beautiful old spot and when spring is really here will be a gem. I believe there is a plan to cultivate all available land within the ramparts, a splendid idea. The convalescent patients will be furnished with helpful exercise and employment and later, with a sufficiency of fresh vegetables for all. I think perhaps this spring we will be allowed to ride our bicycles. It seems very strange indeed that we were not permitted to do so in the fall. However, we are still hopeful. It would give many of us great pleasure and beneficial exercise and I am confident could do no harm.

I have a wonderful picture of your two grandchildren that Helen sent me. Helen is a beauty and Joan, a gem. I do not understand how the mother can think the baby, the lovelier of the two. Helen's perfect little face has created quite a sensation here. What miracles children are! I must write Helen and Jack very soon. I hear from Keith sometimes and he seems to be glad to hear from me. I wonder if Lee is, or has been, near me? So many Canadians have been about and it is possible he is or has been among them. I hope he has my address and I would be very glad of his, and if any of the boys from home, who might have a chance of coming to see me.

I wrote Mr Rigby and hope he received my letter. I trust he is quite recovered from his serious accident. My love to all my friends.

With dearest love, daughter Jane

Pauline has received a fresh letter from her mom and responds immediately. Note that she addresses her mother as "Mammy," and dwells on matters of personal finances, parental health, and the war's end. She is obviously moved by news from home concerning the societal costs of the war. Both "shell shocked" Raine and Frank Goring's disabilities occupy her mind. She is also appalled by the local Conscription Review Board's apparent decision to deprive poor Mrs Styles of her only breadwinner by not exempting her son. As well she has some choice words for Mildred's Bruce—words which were scratched out at a later date. It appears that, after the war, Mildred did think Bruce was "good enough for her" and married him after all.

February 11, 1918
No. 3 Canadian Stationary Hospital, BEF, France

Dearest Mammy,

Your letter of Jan. 13 came today, also one begun by dad and finished by you. It is too bad you have had a fortnight's silence to endure, but perhaps must expect some of our mail to miscarry. You should hear every week and usually twice at least. I think I have received everything sent me in the way of parcels excepting something from Anna and from Jean Burchill. My friends have been most thoughtful. I cannot be grateful enough.

Now before I forget it, without fail, reserve from the $40 a month, the

$26 for uncle Henry as my turn comes around. I am only too happy to do my share, but mammy dear you don't have to consult me about that for it is in your name, and this year after my indebtedness to Guy is paid I want you to consider it yours to do with as you will, to save for a rainy day, or to procure any needed comfort. Next year, 1919 if I am still here I may get Guy to invest it for me as it falls due, that sounds fair. I think an honourable peace will be ours in another year and then it won't be long til I am home. Meanwhile, it is such a comfort to know that you are well this winter. Something tells me that I shall return to find you and dad the dear, courageous, cheerful souls I left behind. You certainly sent me away magnificently and I am more proud of you than I can say, and would be a most unworthy daughter if I did not try to give you some reason to be a little bit proud of me. And after all, surely we are sacrificing less than so very many others. The days we shall have together shall be the richer for this absence.

Dear aunt Celia; I had a letter from her today, I cannot but wonder how Rainie is going to "carry on" successfully with his serious disabilities and Frank! Truly, facing the future with a stout heart must require greater courage than going into battle. And to think that they are only two out of thousands of similar cases.

I am wondering what is to become of poor old Mrs Styles. What pitiful, selfish, wreaks of men sat at that meeting which decreed that her only support be a conscript! They must be soured by their own shortcomings. I am astonished that Bruce is not willing to do his bit and hope that Mildred is not really interested. He is not good enough for her. [The latter two sentences later scratched out.]

Thank you for Louise's address. I shall try to find time to write. Well I have written many times acknowledging the three parcels and the woollens which have kept me so comfy and hope to receive a letter soon telling me that you have heard to that effect.

I am at present on night duty, will be off when you receive this and probably en route to Nice. My love to aunt Caroline, Mildred and Alice. Have you enough coal to keep you warm?

Your own loving daughter, Jane

Five days later, all has changed. Pauline has received a letter telling of her mother's ill health, and she is determined to drop all and return home. She writes her dad that she has put in for "special leave" and is sure there will be no "unnecessary delay."

February 16, 1918
No. 3 Stationary Hospital, BEF, France

Dear Dad,

Just a line this morning before "turning in" after my night of duty. Perhaps today will bring me my "special leave," I cannot get home quickly enough. I know there will be no unnecessary delay. Mammy will get the next note. I know I am going to find her, her old self and we are going to have some wonderful talks. Tell aunt Cass she will have to look to her laurels—I'll wrest them from her, my tongue swings from the middle now.

Oceans of love, Polly

Another five days have passed, and Pauline writes her dad again. Discharge or "special leave"—either one will do, whichever will get her home quicker. She would speak to her sympathetic colonel again that day. Her mind is filled with one thought only: getting home.

February 21, 1918
France

Dear Dad,

Just a line this morning because I am thinking of you and mammy with all my strength. I am going to see Col. Reason again today about my leave or discharge whichever will come through quickest. I cannot think there can be much delay—waiting is intolerable. It seems inconceivable that I am not leaving with this letter—be very sure I shall soon be on my way. I cannot write of other things, only one thing fills my mind—the getting to mammy and you. It is a comfort to know aunt Cass is with you.

Your devoted daughter, Pauline Balloch

Her anxiety is palatable, but progress is being made. News from home has alternatively worried and then calmed her. She will soon be off to England and from there getting back to Canada will not be too difficult.

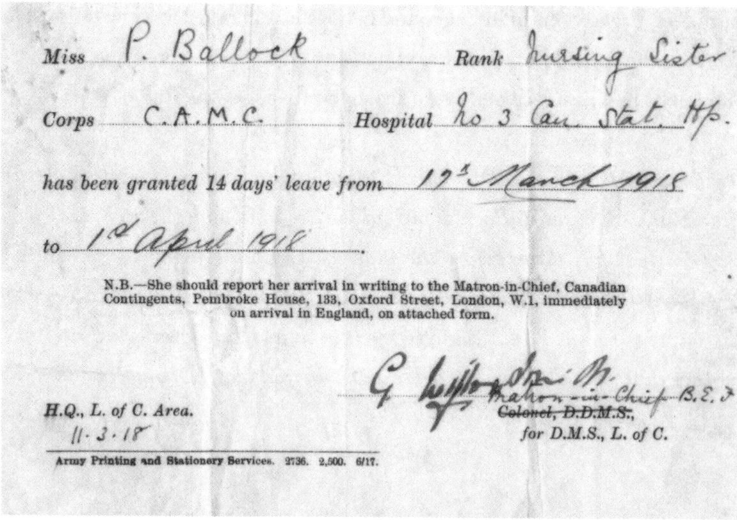

Miss P. Ballock Rank Nursing Sister

Corps C.A.M.C. Hospital No 3 Can. Stat. Hp.

has been granted 14 days' leave from 19th March 1918

to 1st April 1918.

N.B.—She should report her arrival in writing to the Matron-in-Chief, Canadian Contingents, Pembroke House, 133, Oxford Street, London, W.1, immediately on arrival in England, on attached form.

H.Q., L. of C. Area.
11·3·18

G [signature] ~~Colonel, D.D.M.S.,~~ Matron-in-Chief B.E.F.
for D.M.S., L. of C.

Army Printing and Stationery Services. 2736. 2,500. 6/17.

Pauline's initial leave pass, entitling her to go to England on the first leg of her journey home.

February 23, 1918
France
Dear Dad,

I shall soon be en route for England and then it will be an easy matter to secure my transportation to Canada. I cannot express the degree of comfort your second cable has brought me—getting back to you is the one thing for which I wish at the present. Both Matron and Col have been most kind and sympathetic and I think as anxious as I to get me on my way...On the 19th I had a cable from Dr Brown saying "Get discharge—waiting" but I had already put in for leave and believe it will take less time. His cable worried me considerably as it said nothing of mother's condition, but fortunately I had just received word from you that she was stable.

The official War Diary of the Third Canadian Stationary Hospital records that Nursing Sister Balloch departed for England on leave on March 16, 1918—just five days before the massive German spring offensive. All leave was immediately cancelled throughout the British forces all along the Western Front. Pauline had left just in time. Days later, she writes her mother that she has been ordered to pack up and leave Orpington.

March 26, 1918
No 16, Canadian General Hospital, England

Dearest Mammy,

This is just a line written from Orpington to tell you that I have once more been notified to pack my baggage and depart—orders most

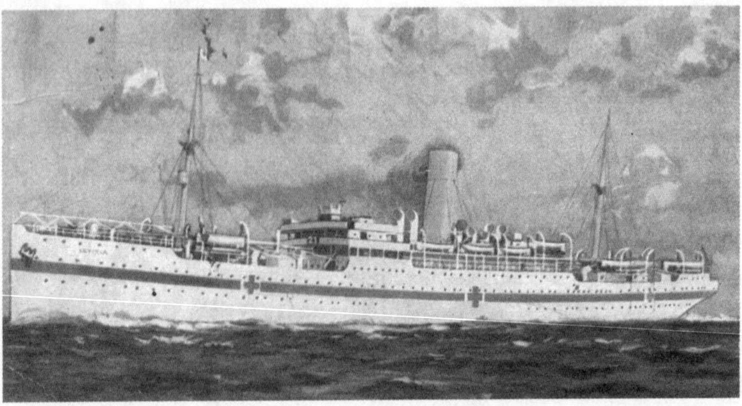

A postcard showing a typical, well-marked, hospital ship, the HMHS Letitia.

happily obeyed for it means I am on my way. I shall mail this just before embarking.

All I can think of is getting home. We shall talk it all out then. Heaps of love to dad and auntie.

Your lovingest, Jane

Pauline's last letter is a historic gem, not for its content, but for its timing and location. She has arrived in Halifax, and is waiting to disembark and catch a train for her parents' home in New Brunswick. The hospital ship she is on is the Llandovery Castle. *Sadly and tragically, the vessel's trips across the Atlantic would be numbered. On June 27, 1918, U-86 torpedoed the clearly marked hospital ship off the coast of Ireland. Convinced it was secretly carrying ammunition, the U-boat captain interrogated survivors from a few lifeboats. Upon realizing his error, he machine-gunned all the survivors. One lifeboat escaped in the fog. Of the 258 persons on board, only 24 survived. All fourteen Canadian nursing sisters died.*

April 7, 1918
Hospital Ship Llandovery Castle, Halifax Harbour

Dearest Mother,

Just time for a line to you to catch the outgoing mail. We won't disembark until Tuesday morning so I can't leave Halifax until the afternoon or evening and as yet know nothing of the trains. There is a possibility that I may not get away from Halifax until Wednesday. However, I will send a telegram to dad from Halifax when leaving so you will not be in doubt.

I cannot get home quickly enough Heaps of love, Pauline

PAULINE D. BALLOCH

Pauline's precipitous return to Centreville in April 1918 to nurse her ailing mother did not end the war for her. Although her mother's health had indeed stabilized by the time Pauline got home, the tragedy of war waged on. On the night of May 30/31, Pauline's former hospital in France, No. 3 Canadian Stationary Hospital, was bombed in a German air raid. Her companion and friend, Dorothy Baldwin, was on duty and was killed by the bomb. Two other nurses, a surgeon, orderlies, and a number of patients were also killed by the explosion. Pauline would have learned of the event through the press. No record of Pauline's shock and grief survive. There is, however, a letter to Pauline from a young nurse, C. A. Ross, who, obviously aware of how close Pauline and "Baldie" had been, wrote her in early June. This letter conveys well the full range of shock and disorientation the bombing caused. Nursing Sister Ross was more than willing to confess that she had been taxed beyond her ability to cope.

No. 2 Canadian General Hospital
France, June 1918

Dearest Balloch,

You will no doubt be surprised to receive a letter from me as I feel quite assured you, right down in your heart, did not expect one. Well dear old girl, it is a great pleasure for me to write, but oh my, it is a sad message I have to give you. I presume you have not heard about it, concerning poor dear Baldie and thought I must write you immediately. I wish I could send you the account in the papers. The calamity occurred Wednesday night or Thursday morning at 12:30 a.m. Darling Baldie was on night duty on the Officers Ward and had just walked into S6 and this awful shell smashed through. P.M. Pringle and dear little MacPherson, one of the dearest girls who ever lived, were killed in the Operating Room. Oh Balloch dear, what a night. We were all under shelter, then in minutes called out. Such a sight we witnessed! You know dear girl, I can't write the details I should love to. I wrote poor Mrs Baldwin and oh how disturbed she will be. We were asked whether we would stay or not, and I, with twenty others, came here [No. 2 Canadian General Hospital]. Ballie dear I couldn't stand it any longer. Bombs all night and shells all day. This is a very nice place. I packed all Baldie's things and left them to be sent home. The poor girl was just awaiting her leave and used to talk to me so much about the time she would have. I couldn't stand that place any longer. I am sitting here with the two Mac Laughlin's and they send their love to you. I feel I haven't a friend in the world. Baldie and I had become very attached. There are just twenty sisters left on the staff. I was in the Operating Room, on day duty, and Pringle (also killed) was at my table. Well old girl how are you? I hope your mother is improving steadily. I am a wreck Balloch. I am of no further use. We have been here ten days and expect to go on duty tomorrow a.m. Our Matron here is Miss Wilson. Also she seems very nice. Col Burne is here also from my home Brockville. Baldie would have enjoyed so much being here. Well old girl I feel horribly upset so will stop. I hope I can see you some day to tell you every particular detail. Good bye for now old girl. Best of love and I know just how you feel when you hear this awful news. Bye Bye, affectionately yours, Charlotte Ross

The war finally did end, and in June 1921, at age forty, Pauline married widower Willard Linwood Carr, age fifty-eight, an arrangement that has more of the ring of practicality than of romance about it. Notwith-

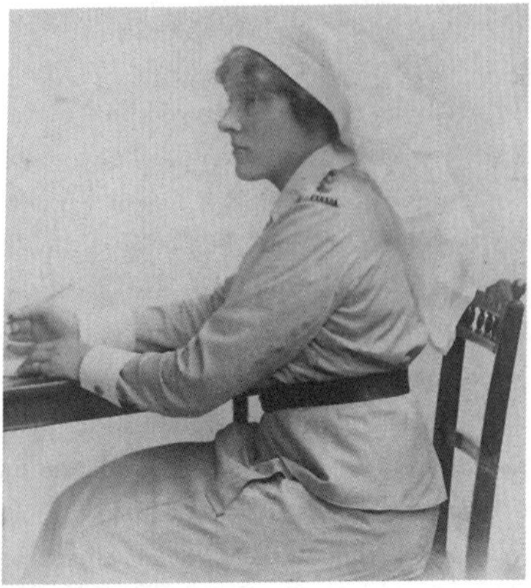

Nursing Sister Dorothy Baldwin, Pauline's good friend, was killed.

standing, sadness would soon intrude upon Pauline's home life. Her father died in August 1921, a few months after her marriage; her mother passed away just over a year later, in October 1922; and a year after that her husband Willard died. Pauline found herself alone. She returned to what she knew: nursing. Moving back to New York City, she worked at St Luke's Hospital. Years later, she returned to Woodstock and functioned there as the highly respected matron of Fisher Memorial Hospital until her retirement. She died at the Carleton Memorial Hospital in Woodstock at the ripe age of eighty-one on August 26, 1962. Her life of service to others had come to a close.

Harry Heckbert

OF SUMMERSIDE, PRINCE EDWARD ISLAND

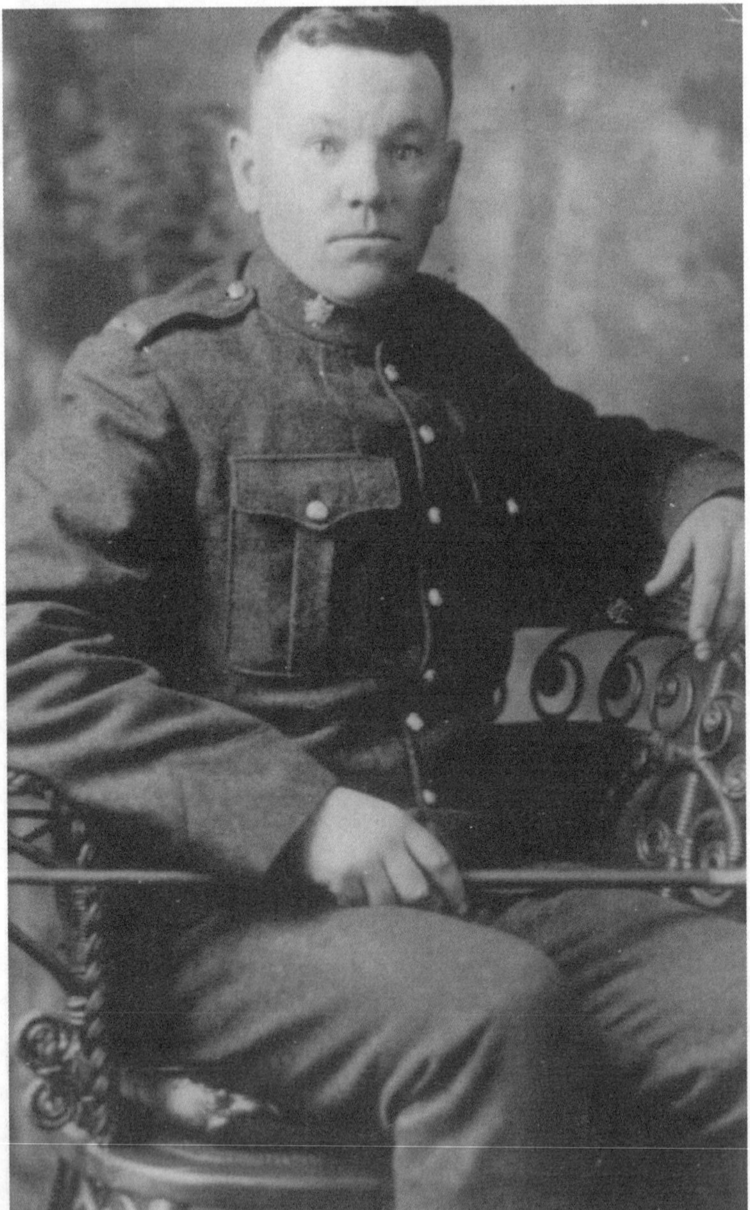

Harry Heckbert in uniform.

Harry Heckbert did not want to go to war. By 1917, the war had raged on for three years. The young, the adventurous, and the unattached had all joined. Harry was rooted. Along with his father Rufus, Harry was a fisherman based in Summerside, Prince Edward Island. After all, were men not needed to work for the cause on the home front as well? He and his dad, along with many other farmers and fishermen, felt they were doing their bit by helping to feed the Canadian war effort. On top of all this, on September 5, 1917, Harry had married the love of his life, Iva Mae Currie. They would soon be welcoming an addition to their family. While Harry and Iva expected a new arrival, the war waited for no one. In the fall of 1917, Harry had been registered for military service, and on March 23, 1918, his active service began. He penned the first of many letters to his wife Iva from Charlottetown.

April 4, 1918
Drill Hall, Charlottetown

Dearest Iva,

This is Wednesday evening and I am kept in tonight and believe me the time seems long here after they all go out. Be sure and come down next week if you can because we can't tell how long we will be here. It is going to be hard to get a pass to go home, but I am just going to ask them once. I did not get the cheque yet and am broke. I was at the station last night and they said they would have it here by tonight and here I am in barracks and I can't get out after it. We have what we call P.T. [physical training] every morning and it is awful hard on my legs. I had to fall out three times already. I played off sick on them today and that is the reason I can't go out tonight. It is awful, I will never get to like it and for two pins I would beat it altogether.

Well darling, I hope you will take good care of yourself for I am thinking about you all the time, Oh honey, when I think of the good times we had together it almost makes me cry, but cheer up honey and don't think about it anymore than you can help. It is awful hard I know, but we never can tell what will turn up. I am totally discouraged and it is no wonder for everybody feels the same here. I am going to wash my towels and knot rags tonight, Wouldn't you like to see me? Ha, ha. I had a cold bath Sunday morning and it was alright. I was examined twice by the doctors since I came down. Every night I get out to have a meal uptown and I can tell you I enjoy it. Oh sweetheart, be sure and come down just as soon as you can. Oh how I would love to see you and give you a big smooch. Well hang, I can't write any more for I feel a big lump coming up in my throat so bye, bye from your own boy.

Yours forever, Pte Harry Heckbert

Harry was not a particularly enthusiastic soldier but he did not stay in Charlottetown for long. His next letter finds him in Amherst, Nova Scotia, on his way to Halifax and then aboard a ship for England. Iva apparently had come to see him before he departed, and they had had a good visit. Tears were shed at their parting, and now the mood of all the troops is glum.

April 14, 1918
Amherst, Nova Scotia

Dearest Iva,

This is Sunday and I am going to try and write you a letter. This is a bum place and everyone feels blue. Well honey, we are under quarantine now and I don't know when we will get out. We can't tell how long we will be staying here. I don't think it will be very long. There was lots of tears shed last night and believe me sweet heart I shed my share. There is some noise here now, a fiddle and piano going all the time. Well honey, write to me soon and let me know how you got home. Tell Flossie [his sister] we had some great fun with her fellow last night. Honey dear, take good care of yourself and don't worry about me too much because I really believe everything will come out all right in the end. But, oh honey, to think that I can't see you now. You must get your picture taken on a postcard and send me one soon because we might get to England any time soon. Oh honey, I can't write any more now so I will have to say good bye for now. With lots of love to everyone. Remember me to all our friends and try and not be too much down hearted but honey dear it is awful hard I know.

Good bye darling for now. Pte Harry Heckbert 3204333 H Coy Amherst N S— I just heard we are going to start for England Monday, I will write as soon as I can.

The news about moving Harry heard proved to be true and by that Wednesday he finds himself in Halifax. He writes to Iva of his trip and of the people he has seen.

April 17, 1918
Halifax

Dearest Iva,

This is Wednesday and we are in Halifax aboard a transport bound for England. They didn't keep us in Amherst very long. I am sitting on my kit bag writing this letter and am using my life preserver as a table. They gave us a great dinner aboard today and I feel fine, don't worry honey too much because something tells me I will be back. There is three big war ships to accompany us over and we will land alright. We have a nice little state room, four of us. I just heard that we will remain here til Friday but it's hard to tell. I will write as soon as I get to Old England and I want you to get Mr and Mrs Newsom's address from Billie (his brother) and send it to me. There are an awful lot of boys aboard. They appear to be a rather jolly lot but a crowd of women on the dock crying make some of them feel pretty bad. When we are marching to the boat I saw that little fellow that used to work in Gallant's drug store, the one that wears the gloves, and when we were at Amherst I saw Andrew Blacquiere. I didn't know him as he is awful thin. Well sweet heart take good care of yourself and be a good girl til your boy returns.

Harry was correct about their imminent departure for England. He writes next from the middle of the Atlantic Ocean. He is beginning to adapt somewhat to his new life, and he has news: he has been appointed to lifeboat guard duty. Although he is at a loss as to why, his background as a fisherman seems the most likely explanation. We also learn why he has been so insistent that Iva "take good care of herself": she is expecting their first child. Harry is an anxious, expectant father going off to war!

April 24, 1918

Sweetheart,

It is Wednesday and we are in the middle of the Atlantic. We are having a great time so far. It isn't very rough so far but it is liable to be so soon enough. We are all kept below. Today for some reason unknown, I have been appointed one of the lifeboat guards and if we get hit with a torpedo I have four minutes to get to my post with my rifle and bayonet. The orders are to bayonet everyone who tries to interfere with the boats while loading. I get clear of all drill on the way over. There is quite a fleet of ships with us and I guess we will get along alright. We are not allowed to say too much about the trip. I feel pretty well, but lonesome for my dear wife, but it will not be for very long honey as I feel pretty sure I shall never get any farther than England. Oh sweetheart, you must take good care of yourself and little Johnny when he comes til daddy gets home. Oh honey, it will be a happy day for me when I land in old Summerside again. I will look forward to the day for I dream of you and home every night. When I get to England and get stationed, so I can give you my address, I would like for you to get your picture taken on a postcard and send to me. I got some taken the night before we left Amherst and paid for them and left your address. The man said he would send them home in case I left before he finished them. When you write, let me know if you get them and if you have one to share, send me one. Well honey, this is after dinner and I feel quite a lot better. The ship is rolling awful though.

It is Thursday afternoon and everything is pretty quiet. We are in the danger zone now and have to keep our life belts with us all the time. This is a great trip sweetheart and one that I will never forget. I think of you and our little home all the time honey. Well sweet, I guess I will bring this letter to a close, be sure and take good care of yourself and be a good girl till your old man comes home. so bye, bye darling.

With lots of love, I remain forever your old man. H. Heckbert

Harry arrives safely in England, and is living at the great training camp at Bramshott, Hampshire, through which tens of thousands of Canadians have already passed. He relates with great zest the excitement of a submarine battle during the crossing and of the sinking of a U-boat just ahead of them. He complains about the food, and states that they are liv-

ing ten men to a tent. He comments on the strange little English houses and their oddly small train compartments—in short, he is adjusting to his new circumstances. As he summarizes matters to Iva, "We are in it and will have to go through like the rest."

April 29, 1918
17th Canadian Reserve Battalion, Bramshott Camp

Hello Honey,

We arrived in England on Sunday morning [April 28] and had quite an exciting trip. The submarines got after us and we sunk three. There was 13 ships of us and we all arrived alright. I was one of the lifeboat guards and we were called up twice, but we arrived alright. This is a queer place, the houses are all brick and very small. We travelled nearly all Sunday night on the train and believe me they go some fast over here. The steamer in front of us sunk one of the German submarines and on arriving at Liverpool, the gunner was presented with 50 pounds and a stripe. We can hear the roar of the guns at the front from here quite plain. We had a nice time on the boat but I think the good times are over now. The grub is bum here. I don't know what they will say for writing this nor care either if they don't like it they can scratch it out. The train cars are awful small here and are divided into little rooms holding eight.

Well sweetheart, I suppose you are worrying quite a lot but it is no use to worry. We will just have to make the best of it for a while. Be sure and take good care of yourself dear. You don't know how often I think of home and you. We are living in canvas tents now, ten men to a tent. We see an odd airship here. If I ever live to get back I will have a lot to tell you. If you intend to send me anything you ought to send it as soon as you can because we can't tell how long we will be here.

You ought to take good care of your money dear for when I get back I will be on the bum. I only got two dollars since I enlisted. You want to watch out and get your share of the fish money. I am going to write Fred [his older brother] after I get time and tell him to do things right. Did you get the letter I sent from Halifax? Well sweetheart, the crowd is pretty downhearted but it isn't awful bad considering it isn't any use to worry now because we are in it and will have to go through like the rest. Well dear, I guess I will have to close for the time. I will write soon again and will be sure to write to me soon.

Bye, bye sweetheart

Harry is still at Bramshott and learning much about army ways. He is seriously unimpressed with the food, poor in quality and scarce. Army pay is small and despite an upcoming leave to Scotland, he worries that his fun will be as limited as his financial resources. He is also wise enough to realize the implications of all the brass on their new uniforms: lots of polishing lies in his future. His thoughts also turn to those at home, to his and Iva's extended families.

May 2, 1918, 17th
Canadian Reserve Battalion, Bramshott Camp

Dearest Honey,

I have a few moments to myself and I think I will try and write you a few lines. Well Honey they work us pretty hard here and we haven't much time to ourselves. The grub is scarce here and we don't get enough to eat. They only give us a pound a month here, that is, four dollars and eighty-six cents and it takes it all to get stuff to eat. If you ever get a chance, send me a few dollars. There are a lot of Summerside boys here. They are going to give us a furlough sometime soon (I don't know how long) ha, ha . A bunch of us are going to Scotland. It won't be much of a time on account of us having no money. Well sweetheart, I hope you are getting along alright and will take good care of yourself til your old man gets home. I wrote you a few days ago but don't know if you will get it or not on account of putting so much news in it. We got our equipment today and there is an awful lot of brass to shine. They keep us going all the time. My legs are getting pretty sore and I can't do them long marches.

I would like if you could send me a box some time with something good to eat. The boys are discouraged here. They don't like it at all and I don't blame them much. How are the fish this spring? and did you get anything out of it yet? How are they all at home? and at your home? How is Tony [Iva's brother] and all the rest? Give my love to them all. How is Gertie [Iva's sister]? I hope she is well and your grandmother? Give my love to them all and don't forget yourself sweetheart. I have to go out a few minutes on parade and will have to close for this time. So bye, bye sweetheart for now, write soon and tell me all the news, yours forever.

Pte H Heckbert 3204333

Harry is concerned about the censorship of his letters, but he need not have worried—nothing was crossed out of his correspondence. He comments on the English countryside, including seeing lots of ducks that his brother-in-law would like to have shot, and on his being broke, or "bum," all the time.

May 4, 1918
Bramshott Camp

Well sweetheart this is Saturday and we have the afternoon off. Earl Reeves[26] and I are up on top of a big hill trying to write some letters. I wrote three before but don't know if you will get them or not on account of things I put in them, for I didn't know the difference til today. They drill us pretty hard, but I like it a little better than I did in Charlottetown. I haven't much news to tell you this time. They won't let us say too much. This is a pretty rough country here, hills rolling and lakes. If Bruce were just here with his gun he would get some great shots, lots of swans in the lakes and ducks too. There is a big lake handy where we drill. They just give us a pound a month here, that is four dollars and eighty-six cents. A fellow is on the bum the whole time. We are in quarantine in camp right now. Well honey, I would just love to see you now. You must get some pictures taken and send me one. Be sure because I want one awful bad. I hope you are well and having a good time. You must take good care of yourself til your old man comes home. Well sweetheart, I guess I will have to say good bye for now. My birthday was yesterday. If you ever get any money you might send me some sometime.

One indication of his homesickness is that Harry writes Iva almost every day. Nonetheless, he is slowly adjusting. He tells her of church parade and asks about planting season back home. He has finally realized that the authorities hold back the men's pay for their own benefit and release it so they can have funds during their leave. One touching indication that you can take the boy out of the Island but not the Island out of the boy is how Harry relates the time difference. He tells Iva not that it is different than in the Maritimes, but that "time is five hours later here than it is on the Island."

26 Earl Reeves (3180368), born Summerside, Prince Edward Island, February 21, 1896; conscripted on November 7, 1917.

May 6, 1918
Bramshott

Dearest Wife,

This is Monday night and I am up on top of a big hill trying to write. I wrote four or five letters before but in case you do not get them I will keep them going. I am pretty well and we are having a fairly good time now but they drill us pretty hard. Well sweetheart, I hope you are well and not too lonesome but cheer up honey, your old man will be home sometime. Oh sweetheart, what a happy day for me when I can land in dear old Summerside. I don't feel as bad as I did first.

How is dear little Gertie and all the rest? I hope your mother and grandmother are all well. Give my love to them all. Where are you staying now? I was just wondering if you were staying home or not. You must take good care of yourself sweet. Are you going to plant any garden this summer? I suppose it won't make much difference for father will look out for us anyway in that line. The time is five hours later here than it is on the Island and when you are getting your dinner we are getting supper here. I wrote some letters before and asked for a few dollars but I don't know if you will get them or not. We don't get any white bread here at all, but we do get lots of rabbit stew. I don't know why they keep our money back, someone said they would give it to us when we went on our furlough, but I don't know whether it is true or not. It is awful to be broke so far from home. All I got was one pound since I came here. Oh sweetheart, I would have just died for one big hug tonight but I will have to wait til I get home. There is some pretty wild boys here but me, oh honey, I am so lonesome sometimes for you I don't know what to do. I will just have to grin and bear it for a while. I was on Church parade Sunday and the first hymn they sung was "Abide with Me." It made me think so much of home I could hardly keep from crying, but I can't act the baby now. I like it a little better than I did, but, oh sweetheart, when I think of you I get sick of the whole business.

All our letters are opened and I can't say much about the trip we had over but when I get back I will have some story to tell. How are they all at home? How is Tony, is he in Summerside yet?

Although not an overtly religious man, Harry's letters are usually on YMCA letterhead. The YMCA of this era was an overtly Christian organization, and keenly interested in the men's spiritual and moral health. Harry tells Iva of going to religious "meetings," which were informal services held in the YMCA huts. He also mentions a lecture they received, most likely from a medical officer (a doctor) about the "temptations" the men would experience while on leave. In reality, this would have been a very blunt talk about prostitutes and STDs that, to say the least, would have made Iva blush, if not leave the room. Harry assures her of his fidelity. Harry also relates seeing some men from home as well as that his camp is on quarantine due to an outbreak of measles and mumps—two very serious diseases in those days.

May 11, 1918
Bramshott Camp

Dearest Wife,

This is Saturday afternoon and a half holiday and I am trying to write you another letter. It is awful warm here now, but the nights are cold. We only had one rainy day since we came here. Well sweetheart, how are you getting along? I hope you are well and all the rest also. We have religious meetings every night, prayers and hymns, all our old hymns. I go every night. If I ever get back it will be no trouble to get me to go to church. I think we are soon going to get on our furlough because yesterday an officer was telling us the things to do and the things not to do. He told us that a greater danger than the battlefield faced us and that was temptation. He meant the girls and women of those cities. But you know what effect that had on me. I will be just the same as before sweetheart and you know what that was. You need never worry about that sweetheart because you know that I mean it and I swear that I will act the man if I am here the rest of my days.

I dreamt about you last night. I thought I was home and little Bridget was there too, but oh honey, when I woke and saw the old tent over my head, a big lump came up in my throat that nearly choked me. I will just have to grin and bear it. How is dear little Gertie? and all the rest? I hope they are all well. Oh sweetheart, I never will forget this if I live to be a hundred years old, but it is no use worrying over it. It makes it all the worse. I would love to get the good old Summerside paper to read. We don't get very much to eat here and I go to bed hungry a good many times and they won't give us our money. I never had a penny for a week. It is awful to be on the bum. I see Lyle Robinson and Harold and Claude Leard[27] every day and I saw Kingsley Grady[28] the other day. He is quite a big man now. This is a kind of quarantine camp here now. We will have to stay here sometime yet for there is measles and mumps here. My legs are pretty sore this afternoon and I don't believe I will ever stand the long marches.

A flock of swans just flew past on their way to the lake. We have moving pictures and concerts every night. Some of them are pretty good. They are all free. It is a good job for there wouldn't be many there if they charged much. The boys are laying around everywhere asleep. I was on the Island's tug of war the other night and we hauled the other fellows all over the place. Oh honey don't forget to get your picture taken and be

---

27 Both Harold Leard (3204250), born 1891, and Claude Leard (3204145), born 1895, had been living in Summerside at the time of their conscription.

28 Kingsley L. Grady (522104) joined in November 1915 at Halifax. but due to health reasons appears to have been employed at Bramshott Camp.

sure to send me one for I will be waiting every mail for one. I won't say anything in this letter about wanting money because I guess I said it in every other letter.

Oh honey dear, I will have to say bye once more, Harry

Harry tells Iva about PT, which the troops have dubbed "Physical Torture." Upon entry into the army, most men were not sufficiently fit or at least sufficiently hardened to the tough physical demands of infantry life on the Western Front. Long marches wearing a pack ranging in weight from forty to sixty pounds and carrying a rifle were to become part of Harry's future. He had to be built up into sufficient shape to endure such demands.

May 14, 1918
Bramshott Camp

Dear Wife,

This is Tuesday evening and I thought I would write you a few lines to let you know how I am getting along. I didn't work very hard today. I was to see the doctor this morning and I got clear of PT for a few days. I suppose you wonder what PT is. It is an exercise called Physical Training that the boys here call Physical Torture. My knees are pretty sore, the doctor says rheumatism is getting right after them and I shouldn't wonder if I should be turned down with them yet. Well sweetheart, we are getting a little better acquainted with the place here and like it a little better now. If they would only give us a little more to eat it would be much better. Everyone is broke here and it is no wonder, they use us pretty mean. About paying us, all I got yet was one pound.

Writing his next letter, Harry is in the hospital—nothing serious, just a sore throat, but he does not mind the break. He relates an incident he found funny, and asks about the separation allowance which Iva is to receive from the Dominion government. He also mentions the herring money that is Harry's and Iva's share of the income from the family fishing business.

May 24, 1918
Bramshott Camp

This is a holiday here. Don't get scared when I tell you I am in the hospital with tonsillitis. My throat is just a little sore, that's all. I will soon be out again. I have a great rest. I just heard this morning that it was reported around Summerside that the ship we came across on was lost. I hope you were not very scared sweetheart. No honey, we are not lost yet. My rheumatism is getting worse all the time here. I had to fall out of parade the other day with it. You know we just have four blankets to sleep on and no tick either and that is great for rheumatism. I am expecting a letter every day but don't know when I will get one. My chum Ben is in the hospital too with mumps. Well honey, I suppose you will think it is bull when I tell you I never had a drink of any kind of liquor since I left Amherst except a few drinks of beer and very few at that, but it is the truth sweetheart. I try not to think so much of home but the thoughts of you and our little home makes it too hard to forget. They feed us a little better in the hospital and believe me I am glad that I am here. About the first thing that made me laugh since I came here happened yesterday right alongside of our hospital tent. There was the doctor's big tent. There was an awful squall came and I just happened to look out when I saw the tent start down the valley, three or four doctors in it and thousands of medical sheets and medicine bottles and tables and everything. Believe me it was going some! I nearly died laughing. Did you get any separation allowance yet? I hope you did get it alright. Did you make anything out of the herring this spring? If you can ever spare me a dollar or two please send it and I will assure you it will not be wasted no matter how little it is.

I guess I will have to close for this time as I have to go and have my throat swabbed out. Bye, bye sweetheart with a million kisses and a love that no one knows but ourselves.

I remain yours forever, your old man

Harry is still homesick, and is off to church again. He relates a touching story of how, during service, he recalled Iva's voice singing the same familiar hymn and it brought him to tears. He is also meeting a great number of men he knew from the Summerside area. Even his PT instructor, who was twice wounded earlier in the war and had once been buried alive by shellfire, is an acquaintance of Harry's brother Bruce.

June 2, 1918
Bramshott Camp, England

My Dear Wife,

This is Sunday afternoon and Dwight and I are under some trees writing letters. It is terrible hot here today. Well sweetheart, how are you these times? I hope you are well and happy and are not worrying too much. I am pretty well myself but I worry a lot about you dear. I just can't help it. You know how it is dear. Oh honey, if I ever get back no more soldiering for me. I was at church today. We had a minister from London. He was a dandy. The other night I was in "the tent" where we sing and they sung all the old hymns I knew and it made me feel terrible lonesome. When they sang "son of my soul" I could hear your voice so plain singing the last verse that it brought the tears to my eyes. You know you often used to sing it around the house. Joe Gillis[29] is here now. I see him every evening and Maynard Sonier[30] too. I met a fellow last night that used to work at Matthews and Dick Clarks. He came up to me and said "hello Heckbert." I didn't know him at all. His name is Williams. Andrew Arsenault[31] from Ross Corner is here. He is a PT instructor. He has been wounded twice. Bruce and all the rest know him, be sure and tell him.

I was to the doctor yesterday and got clear of PT drill for another week. I never got any letters from you yet and I must have written about fifteen to you and the old man, father, I mean, but I am expecting one every day. They feed us a little better these days but we don't get enough yet. It seems just like a dream to me to be here. What drill I learn in one day I forget it the next. How is everyone home? I would love to see them all now. How is your mother and grandmother and all the rest? Tell Gertie I often think of her. Tell her when I come home I will bring her something nice. I suppose Tony is gone away before this. I got two letters the other day that came to Amherst after we left; one from Willie and Papa. There is an awful lot of bicycles in this country, almost every girl drives one. Are you staying at home or in at our home? I often wonder. Oh sweetheart, if I just could get home before you become a mother I would be satisfied but that is impossible. It is too bad and when I think of it, it near breaks my heart. Well dear, I guess this is all the news for this time and with a million kisses and all my love, I remain your old man forever.

Pte H. H. 3204333

Harry still has not received a letter from Iva. This delay in transatlantic mail service was beginning to wear on Harry's nerves, but he persisted

29 Joseph L. Gillis (3181671), born in Summerside, Prince Edward Island, 1897.
30 Maynard Sonier (3181640), born in Summerside, Prince Edward Island, 1899.
31 Andrew Arsenault (69031), born in Bedeque, Prince Edward Island, 1896; joined up in November 1914 and served with the 26th Infantry Battalion.

in writing home. He relates seeing more men he knew, expresses his hopes of one day obtaining leave for Scotland, and asks for some money from home for that purpose. He also tells of his difficulties in marching long distances and of a visit to a fish market which made his mouth water, especially the sight of lobsters. Finally, he tells Iva of "tin town," a series of little buildings just outside camp erected by English merchants. Although very convenient, such establishments had a reputation for being pricey, and were geared to relieve the soldiers of their money as soon as they left camp.

June 9, 1918
Bramshott Camp

My Darling Lonesome Wife,

This is Sunday afternoon and I am about a mile from the camp. I never got a letter yet and am awful lonesome. I heard that some Canadian mail came in today. We moved to our reserve the other day and we have huts to live in now, about 30 men to a hut. I met Gordon Arbing[32] the other day and he is pretty well and Brad Beers too, he is an officer. I was out on an eight mile march the other day and managed to make it alright. We are going on one this week with our packs on and I bet it will get my goat. I visited three little towns yesterday afternoon and stopped at a fish market and saw a lot of lobsters and believe me they made my mouth water. I didn't have one cent either but when I get some I will certainly go back. I was expecting some from home but the mail is terrible slow. Well sweetheart, I would love to know how you are getting along

32 Gordon Arbing (111104), born in Bedeque, Prince Edward Island, 1885; joined the 6th Regiment, Canadian Mounted Rifles, in Amherst, Nova Scotia, in April 1915.

and how you feel? I hope you are well and not too lonesome but I know how it is and it worries me quite a lot. They don't give us very much to eat and I am hungry nearly all the time. Oh sweetheart, if I could only get home when our dear baby is born I would be satisfied but that is impossible. Cheer up dearie. I know everything will come out alright in the end. There is a little town by the reserve called "tin town" and it is Tin Town alright. They charge three times for everything.

If I ever get my pass I am going to Scotland and I hope to get a little money from home first. I hope you get your separation allowance alright. Did Papa get the deed made out for our place yet? If I could only hear from you once in a while I would feel a lot better. We are so far apart that it takes a long while for mail to get here. But you must write me a lot of letters so they will be coming all the time. Did you get any pictures taken yet? If you didn't you better get busy or I will be mad (ha, ha) I am going to have some taken here sometime if I ever get the price. Did you get the ones I got taken in Amherst? I bet I loomed up like you know what I mean. I saw a girl the other day that looked an awful lot like you and my heart came up in my mouth. I thought that you followed me over here (ha, ha) I am going down to see Andrew Arsenault this evening. I haven't seen him yet. Some of our boys were down to Witley Camp yesterday afternoon and saw the King. They say they had a great time. Did they get Billy, Earl and Joe yet? I hope they will never have to come. I often look up at the sun and wonder if you are looking at it too. Some of the boys here hardly ever think of home and never write, but I never can get it out of my mind. Well dearest, I guess I will have to close for this time. So wishing you all kinds of good luck and a million kisses and you know how much I love you dear. I will close once again.

From your old man, forever to the dearest wife a man ever had

Harry finally receives his first letter from Iva. His thoughts return to home again and to matters financial, the "fish money," the separation allowance, and, if there is any to spare, a few bucks for him in case he gets leave. Not all has been well at the camp, however. The Canadian troops, already with a reputation for pushing back if discipline is too strict, had rebelled and rioted, destroying the "clink" or jail where severely disciplined troops were placed. Harry reports casualties, including deaths.

June 20, 1918
17 Reserve Battalion, Bramshott Camp

Dear Wife,

I received a letter yesterday and was very glad to hear that you are all well at home. I am pretty well and they isn't working us so hard now. You said you sent me a parcel but I didn't get it yet. Earl and I are in the Salvation Army writing room, writing letters. Some of the first draft boys are going on their pass tomorrow, but we haven't heard anything about ours yet. If you don't get the separation money you must write to Ottawa about it because you are entitled to it. Did you get any money from the fishing this Spring? I am going to write to Fred about it. It rained all day here and we didn't drill any but they will take it out on us some other time. I hope you will send me a little money soon and some socks too. When I told you to try and save some money I didn't mean to go without things you need. I meant that if you did well out of the fish to lay a little aside for a rainy day, but I know it costs a lot to live now.

They are awfully strict here and they keep us shining brass nearly all the time. We are in the R.C.R.'s [Royal Canadian Regiment] and they are noted for that. Well honey, I would love to be in Summerside tonight. I suppose I would make a run for Gallant's drug store first things (ha, ha) Well I don't know that I would, I would be so glad, I wouldn't know what to do. I hope you isn't working too hard these days for you know you must take care of yourself now. Did you put in any garden this Spring? If you ain't got any chow for me when I come home you will catch it. There was quite a scrap in camp here and some of them croaked and some more in the hospital all broke up. They had some time. They tore the guts out of the clink. Well dear, I guess this will be all for this time. So hoping you are well, I will say bye, bye dearest, love to all.

Yours forever, your old man Pte H. H.

Harry has been on a route march with his pack, and he didn't like it. In fact he had to drop out and then report to the doctor. He hopes his rheumatism will ensure he is not fit enough for France. Iva must have related a story of "morning sickness," which Harry refers to as her being "sick." He tries to be patient awaiting the arrival of his parcel, his few dollars, and a picture of Iva. All these things will take time.

June 23, 1918
England

My Dear Wife,

I just received your letter about an hour ago and was very glad to hear that you are well. I am pretty well too dear—oh the rheumatism! I was out on a route march yesterday with a pack on and I flopped when I got a couple of miles out. I went to the doctor's office this morning but he wasn't in and I am going again in the morning. I knew I couldn't go far with all that old guts on my back. I never got any parcels, but I am expecting some every day. I hope you can send me a few cents before long for it is awful to be without a cent you know. I don't mean for you to send me money every time I write for it but I have been here quite a while and didn't get any yet.

I know you will need about all you can get to live on but your old man needs a little dear. I know you will send some as soon as you have any to spare. I don't think I will ever go to France on account of my stiff joints. I am sitting on a hill here all alone and I tell you honey I am pretty lonesome. Oh sweetheart, if I could only be home when you are sick I would be satisfied but it is pretty hard to get out of the army now, but I have a pretty good case but I am going to try and work it too. The whole business just seems like a bad dream, but it is no dream is it dear? It is too real.

Now honey you promised to send me a picture but I never got it yet. Perhaps I am expecting it too soon but I can't help it dear. It was foolish of me to come away in the first place without it anyway. I wish you could send me Allan's address so I could write to him. Bruce [Harry's younger brother] must have a pretty bad hand and he must find it hard to hug Adeline (ha, ha) Is Zilla out home yet? If she is tell her I am going to bring a nice soldier home with me for her for I know that is just what she wants. I hope they will have the luck that she wished us on that post card she sent us last winter (ha, ha) I know she won't be mad when you tell her what I said. I hope your mother and all the rest are well and dear little Gertie too. Give them all my love and tell your grandmother I hope to get out of this business before winter and that I expect to see them all again.

I guess I will have to close for this time and with a million kisses and ten bushels of love, I remain yours forever, your old man Pte H. H.

Harry's falling out during route march has gotten him into hot water. For not asking permission of an officer first, he was punished by having to do extra drill. He is also to appear before a Medical Board, which will determine his fitness status. Harry hopes he does poorly—perhaps he'll even be sent back home. He has much to learn, however, about the Canadian army's need for men in the summer of 1918. This need includes thousands of men far behind the front line in jobs in support of the fighting troops. Still no parcel, no picture, and as for the name of their child, he will defer to Iva's judgment. On the good news side, Harry has received his pay, and what does the boy from the Island do? He buys food—including a can of sardines, apparently Harry's favourite.

June 27, 1918
England

My Dear Wife,

This is Thursday and I am off parades until I go up for a Medical Board. I was out on a march the other day with a pack on and I only went about two miles and dropped out. I got into trouble over it too. I should have asked permission from an officer to fall out but I didn't know the difference. I had to do four extra drills with the pack on but I went to the doctor again and now they have me up for a board. I hope they turn me down and then I will be home to my dear wife again. Well honey, I am thinking about you all the time and worrying a lot too. I can't help it, I hope you are well and not worrying too much. How are they at home? Oh how I would like to walk in on you all today. Tell Gertie I expect she will be after the fellows by the time I get home. I hope your mother, grandmother and all the rest are well. I got your letter the other day and didn't have time to answer til today. I suppose everything is on the bum now in Summerside but believe me hon, it is good enough for me still, and, God knows, I might be there before long if this examination turns out all right. I don't know when I will get it but they won't catch me asleep anyway. I am glad that I got clear of drilling for a while anyway. I saw Joe Gillis today. He arrived at the Reserve the other evening and Maynard Sonier too. They laughed when they saw me doing pack drill and it was no wonder. I am glad you didn't see me (ha, ha). Well sweetheart, I am very much disappointed about the picture because I wanted it oh so bad and you would have been alright too. I am awful mad about it. I will beat your bum when I get home. You must get a nice name for that little fisherman when he arrives. You know that I will like any name that you do. Do you think you will go to the hospital? I think it will be better for you but you can use your own judgement. Oh sweetheart if I could only get home, wouldn't that be great? You know they won't take a man to France unless he is a whole man and you know that I ain't all here.(ha, ha) How is your grandmother? I hope she is well and happy but I suppose there is something worrying her all the time. Tell Lee I think she is getting old and if she likes I will bring her a nice soldier home when I come for I know she likes soldiers (and their guns). They paid us last night and believe me I had some scoff, even a can of sardines. Did you send me any money? If you did I didn't get it or any parcels. A lot of the boys got parcels but your poor old man got none. I got two pairs of socks last night but they are not much good.

I guess I will have to say bye, bye once more so with a million kisses and ten bushels of love, I am your forever, your old man Harry.

Dominion Day in France, July 1, 1918, was a historic occasion for the Canadian Corps, tens of thousands of whose soldiers celebrated the event with large-scale, highly competitive sporting events. Harry Heckbert was there. He describes some of the impressive scene, including the thousands of men sitting on the hillside watching the events. Harry also reports on what he assesses as the large-scale marital infidelity, which he sees all around him during such public gatherings, and once again assures Iva of his loyalty. Nonetheless, Harry is also enjoying himself. Temporarily placed on cookhouse duty awaiting his Medical Board hearing, he is eating well. He tells Iva of enjoying an entire jar of pickles all by himself.

July 1, 1918

Hello Sweetheart,

It is Dominion Day and a holiday here. They have quite a programme of sports for the boys but I am working in the cookhouse yet and believe me I am feeding my face these days. I wrote you three letters this last four days, don't think I am crazy honey but I get so lonesome I just have to write. The boss of the cookhouse came in at dinner time and told us there was a bucket of beer for our table at suppertime. That will be some treat. I haven't much news this time, but I had to write something. I went and signed for my pass last night but I don't know whether they will give me one or not on account of being up for a board but I am trying anyway. If I get it I am going to Edinburgh, Scotland. I thought I would have had a dollar or two from you by this time but I suppose you are like me, you have none to spare hon. I know you will have a hard enough time to get along till your old man gets home but it may not be very long before I am in Canada. I wish they would put me up for board soon so I would know what I am going to get. B 3 classification goes back to Canada. I hope I will be B12 (ha, ha).

Oh Honey, if you were just here this afternoon you would see some grand sights. I am sitting on the side of a big hill all alone and the whole hillside is dotted with girls and soldiers and they are having a great time, but I have to stay alone. I am looking ahead to the time when I go home and can look my sweetheart in the face and say I have been true to you, sweetheart, but there are lots of married men here that I know and I often see them with the girls. It is awful for that around here. You must write to me often honey and let me know how you are because I am all the time wondering if you are well and I expect a letter every time the mailman comes. I never got any parcel yet. When you write tell me all the news and don't forget to write often. I sure have a snap [a good job] now and I was just thinking it was too good to last long. I got into a big jar of pickles today and I eat so many I got a pain in my side (ha, ha). Tell Lee

I see Joe everyday and he is well and appears to enjoy soldering alright. I expect when I leave the cookhouse I will be so fat that I can't drill any more. Oh sweetheart give my love to them all at home and remember me to them all in Summerside. I guess I will have to sign it off.

Here's hoping this finds you well and happy, bye, bye sweetheart, forever yours, your old man.

Harry appeared before the Medical Board on July 2. His complaint was officially recorded as pains in his hips, knees, and shoulder which interfered with his ability to participate in regular parade. He lost his mess house position and was moved to the Convalescent Depot a short distance away. He would be there for about a month. As a result, he lost his chance to go on leave, but he again meets a familiar face from the Island: Calvin M. Chappell, a farmer from Summerside. He tells Iva of receiving her parcel and of his sharing it with Cal. He also admits to having forgotten his wife's birthdate. One imagines that his talk of their soon-to-arrive child did not entirely lessen Iva's ire at hearing this tidbit of forgetfulness.

July 7, 1918
England

Dearest Wife,

This is Sunday afternoon and awful hot. I got your parcel Friday evening and believe me I had an awful scoff. I was up for Board and was transferred to the C.C.D. [Canadian Convalescent Depot]. That is a place where all men go when they come out of the hospital before they go back on drill again. I am having a pretty good time and haven't got to work very hard. Well sweetheart, I often wonder how you are these days. I hope you are well and happy but it is hard to be happy these days, isn't it? Dear, Cal Chappell[33] is here too in the same hut as me. The other night one of the fellows in the next hut to ours cut his throat, but he didn't die. They took him to the hospital. All our boys went on pass Friday but I didn't go on account of being in the C.C.D. but I will go later. I was awful glad to get the socks and the other stuff as well. Some of the apples spoiled but the chicken and cakes were swell. I haven't had a letter from you for a week but I heard there was a big Canadian mail in today and I expect some tomorrow. Did you send me any money yet? If you did I didn't get it yet. If you ever send me any I think it would be just as well to send it in two or three letters. Don't put it all in one so if one got lost it wouldn't be so bad. I am awfully disappointed about your picture and am right sore about it. I was to church this morning and it made me feel awful especially when he prayed for "all our loved ones at home." I tell you sweetheart it almost brought the tears.

Well sweetheart when do you expect the little fisherman? I expect it won't be very long now before he arrives. I will have to celebrate when I get the news. When is your birthday hon? I have forgotten the date! I ought to be ashamed of myself but I am awful absent minded. Cal Chappell got a parcel today and we went out on the grass and had a dandy scoff. We have to pass anything like that around you know, but when I get some lobster I will beat it to the woods alone.(ha, ha). It costs an awful lot to send parcels don't it? You don't know how it cheers a fellow up when he gets one. When I get my pay I am going to send you some souvenirs; badges and other little things. I am collecting badges now and have quite a lot of nice ones.

When I went before the doctors one of them said he couldn't see anything wrong with me and wanted to send me back to drill, but our Medical Officer said they would throw me out first day, so they sent me down here. It is about half a mile from the Reserve Battalion base. I am getting two nice sets of teeth soon. I told him to make them out of cast iron so I

33 Calvin M. Chappell (3204325), born in Summerside, Prince Edward Island, 1890; conscripted in March 1918 along with Harry.

could eat the old tools. He laughed until I thought he would split. I think I will write to father today if I don't get too lazy. That job in the cook-house didn't last long but it was good while it lasted. Frank Lyle[34] is here at the C.C.D. but I didn't see him yet. I am going to hunt him up tonight. Don't forget to send your old man a little bit of money when you can spare it. Did you get the separation money yet?

I guess this will be all for this time, so give my love to all and good bye sweetheart with a million kisses and all kinds of love, I am your old man forever. Write soon.

Harry is now a happy man. Not only has he received three letters from Iva at once; he has also received the money order. The very first thing he does to celebrate is go to the store and buy more sardines. How he enjoyed that scoff!

July 15, 1918
England

My Dear Wife,

I received the money order today and believe me it just came in time because I was hungry. The first thing I done was go into a store where they sold good stuff to eat. I got two cans of sardines and a lot of other stuff and believe me I had some scoff. When I got my belly full I came to the Salvation Army hut to write you. Well sweetheart, I got three letters from you today and was very glad to hear that you are very well. I got a

34 Frank Lyle (257777), born in St. Eleanor's, Prince Edward Island, 1893; conscripted in Saskatoon, January 1918.

scare when the corporal handed me the telegram. I was scared to open it but when I got it opened I wasn't very scared. I am down at the C.C.D. yet and am not working very hard. I don't know how long they will keep me here before they send me up to the Reserve Base. Well honey, I am sending you a couple of cards. I hope you like them. I am going to send you some souvenirs when I go up town. I had a letter from father today and one from Billie and Earl [his brothers] and Joe. So I have to spend the evening answering them. I got the pictures alright. They turned out pretty good. I certainly haven't got so much fat on now as I had then. How are they all home there? There is never a day passes but I think of them all and you. Oh hon if I just could see you tonight! What a meeting it would be.

Harry worries about Iva and the due date of their baby. He admits he's a worrier, and again tells her how lonesome he is. His stress must have been obvious, for his chum Andrew Arsenault distracts Harry by taking him out to a museum in a nearby town. Harry is amazed by all the things he sees. Still, Harry's greatest distraction is food. He continues to spend the money Iva sent him. This time it is pickles, sardines, and even a can of salmon. Another memorable feed!

July 24, 1918

My Dear Wife,

This is Wednesday evening and I am awful lonesome and anxious to know how you are by this time. I haven't got any letters for about a week except two that I got from sister Lena. Oh hon, if I could only know that everything is alright I would feel more contented because I worry more or less all the time. I can't help it dear. You don't know how I feel sometimes and I couldn't begin to tell you but I will hope and pray for everything to be alright sweetheart. I dodged off parade this afternoon and had a good sleep in the woods. I dreamed I was home in your place and I thought I was drunk and your grandmother gave me an awful lecturing. I had to laugh when I woke and thought it over, funny wasn't it. When I get word that you are alright and it is over I think I will have to celebrate (ha, ha) No hon I will behave myself as long as I am here but I will feel a lot better after I find out the news.

I was up to Hazelmere with Andrew Arsenault Sunday afternoon and he took me to the museum. Oh sweetheart, if you could just see the things that I saw there. There was everything imaginable. I saw a crab with claws about four feet long and all kinds of fish stuffed and animals of all kinds also snakes and birds and plants. Also old coins and human skulls and Indian bows and arrows and fish spears and nets and tomahawks and shells. I couldn't begin to tell you one quarter of the things I seen there. Andrew had a hard time to get me out. I am going to go back next Sunday. Oh if I could just take my sweetheart to see all the things there. How nice it would be. I thought I would get over being lonesome but I never will as long as I am away from my darling wife, which I hope won't be long. They are giving the Germans the devil now; everything looks pretty good these days. Do you hear from Allan very often? I would love to have his address so I could write to him. I believe I got fat since I got that money. I certainly had some awful feeds. I went down the street the other night and bought a bottle of pickles and two cans of sardines and a can of salmon and biscuits and went into the woods and cleaned up the whole business, pickles and all! Believe me, I was some full. It made me think of home to have a full belly. How are they all at home? Is Tony at Borden yet? How is your grandmother and all the rest ? Gertie I suppose is growing like a weed. I expect she will have a fellow when I get back. Oh, but I don't know, she may not take after her big sister after all (ha, ha). Well sweetheart, I guess I will have to close for this time. So hoping everything is alright with you and you are well.

I will say bye, bye and God bless my darling, love forever, your old man

HARRY HECKBERT

Knowing that Iva's due date is near, Harry worries all the time. Another parcel and a blowout of eating help little. While there is much preaching about sexual temptations, Harry assures Iva again that he stands firm. Still, he intimates that, upon his return, there will be a great deal of kissing and hugging to make up for lost time. He further confesses that, although he would like the government to give up on him as simply an expense, for the first time he alludes to the possibility of his actually going to France.

July 31
Bramshott Camp, England

My Dear Wife,

This is Wednesday and I have the day off after being up all night. I am awful anxious to hear from you and expect a telegram any day now. Oh sweetheart, I wish I were just home with you where you are for it would be a lot easier for you. I worry a lot about you lately, I can't help it dear. Although I know you will be looked after alright I can't help worrying. Oh hon, when this awful war is over and I get back to my darling wife, it will be like going to heaven, won't it dear? I am so lonesome today I don't know what to do. If I only knew you were alright I would be more content. I ain't working very hard these days, but the boys tell me I am getting thin. I always get thinner in the summer anyways.

I got a box from home yesterday and had a great blowout. Oh hon, it cheers me up to think that I am not forgotten over here. I know this trip won't hurt me any and it will be all the better when I get home. It will be like starting all over again. I will have to kiss and hug an awful lot to pay up for all the lonesome days I am putting in now. When I think how happy we were together and having to leave my darling to come away over here, I couldn't begin to tell you how I feel. After I get back I suppose I will forget all about it. Our boys will soon be going to France but they haven't got anything on me yet. I guess it will be sometime before I go (ha, ha). They will find out some day that I am just a bill of expense to the government and let me go. It isn't the work or fighting that worries me, it is being away from you so long and if I wasn't married I wouldn't care a rap! It is altogether different now because I want to get back to my dear little wife and kiddie as quick as possible. They preach about temptations an awful lot over here but my love for you dear is strong enough to overcome any temptation. There is no danger whatever of me being tempted. All I have to do is to think of you and I can overcome anything. Well dear I guess I will have to close for this time so hoping you are well as can be expected.

I am forever your old man

Rainy weather, a lack of mail, and the anxiety of not knowing all get Harry down in spirits. He tells Iva how lonely he is. He recalls how choked up he became when they parted on the train platform back on the Island, and he wishes he could be home. This is especially the case now, for, as he not so tactfully reminds her, she is "sick"—that is, soon to give birth. Despite Harry's ignorance as to the subtleties of pregnancy, his heart is in the right place.

August 1, 1918
Bramshott Camp

My Dear Wife,

This is Thursday night and it is raining to beat the band. I only got two letters in these last two weeks and the way you are makes me worry quite a lot. If only I could get more letters, but the mails are all bunged up and some days I will get a whole bunch. I would love to get one tonight saying everything is alright. You said you would telegraph and I have been looking for it for a week. Well Dearie, I do hope it is all over by this time and when you get able you must write me some letters. I don't care how many, a whole arm full if you can. You don't know how I feel when I get a letter from you. Oh Dearie, if I could just be near you when you are sick it would be great to be back. I will never forget, on the station platform, when I said goodbye, a lump came up in my throat and when I went in the car I couldn't speak. Sweetheart, when I get home I'll guarantee I never will leave again. I am awful lonesome tonight. I hope you isn't as lonesome as I am dear, but I know it is hard for you to get along without me. We all have our troubles in this world, but surely this war will soon be over and then dear, Oh hon, what a big hug you will get.

Did you get your money yet? You must have got some when you sent me that. It is just about all gone now. I tried to get my pass when I had the money but I couldn't. I will have to wait until I get up to the Reserve Base and then I won't have any money. There is a big dance here Monday night in the mess room and the officers told us we could bring our lady friends. Not for me, I never go to anything like that and I can't enjoy anything without you dear. Lots of the married men will have girls that night alright. I will turn in and have a sleep. I haven't much more news for this time. I wrote to Mrs Burns and uncle Charlie today. I guess I will have to say bye, bye dear. With a million kisses and ten bushels of our love.

I am your forever, Harry. Please write as soon as you can and give the little fisherman a great big kiss from me.

Harry writes again the very next day, and the reason is clear: despite their plans, Iva still hasn't cabled Harry with any news. Moreover, his chum Cal has received a cable, and it is bad news: his wife is fine but their baby died. This stirs Harry's nerves considerably, but to his credit he is moved with compassion for his chum and the grief of his wife back on the Island.

August 2, 1918

Hello Sweetheart,

Although I wrote you a letter yesterday I had to write another today as I am awful lonesome. Every time I go to church I get lonesome. It makes me think of the time you got me started to go first. Well sweetheart, you said you would send me a cablegram when the little man arrived. I hope you will dear. I am expecting it every day now. Cal Chappell got one from his wife last night and it said, "child dead, mother well." Oh hon, it started one thinking. Poor Cal, he isn't a bad soul. Him and I chum around a lot together and I tell you hon he thinks a lot of his wife, but he don't think as much of her as I do of mine. All the same, he is a good boy over here and I like him fine. I do hope dear that everything is alright.

Another Sunday, another church service and another sermon, but this was a great one! Still lonesome, Harry worries about Iva's being "sick," and informs her that the money she sent is all gone. It appears, however, that Harry spent the remainder of it in an attempt to cheer up his poor depressed chum Cal by treating him to a feast of eggs, bread, and cake. Harry clearly has a kind heart.

August 4, 1918
Bramshott Camp

My Dear Wife,

This is Sunday and I just got back from church and no mail so I thought I would write a few lines before dinner. Well dear this is the lonesomest morning I spent for a long while and I am so anxious to hear from you that I am worrying quite a lot. I know it is no use worrying, but I can't help it hon, to think that you are sick and I am so far away. This is the fourth anniversary of the war and the preacher preached a great sermon today. Well hon, that money is all gone now that you sent and I am on the bum once more. I wrote Uncle Charlie and Mrs Burns the other day. I don't know how many letters I wrote to you this week, I guess one nearly every day hon. I do hope and pray that everything will be alright and I would give a good bit to know right now. Poor Cal took it pretty hard, he didn't get up for breakfast at all today. I felt sorry for him. We went down to a restaurant today and had four eggs apiece and bread and cake and two cups of tea apiece—some chow-out.

Well sweetheart, I guess I will have to close for now.

Bye, bye with a million kisses and ten bushels of love, I remain forever, your old man, Hal. Write soon sweetheart—I just wrote Mrs Newsham.

Harry receives a letter from Iva, but given the six-week-or-so mail delay, it is from the time just before she entered the hospital. He is distressed to hear that she is broke, and wonders how that can be. He threatens to write a stiff letter to his brother Fred, who appears to be the one in change of Harry's share of the fishing enterprise. He even pledges to sell his gear to help Iva out, but by the end of the letter reconsiders, for that would leave him helpless upon his return. He realizes his child must be born by now, notwithstanding the lack of a cable to that effect. He ends his letter by wishing that Iva give little "Johnny" a hug from him. Harry clearly has his heart set on a son.

August 9, 1918
Bramshott Camp

My Dear Wife,

I just received your letter, the first I got for about two weeks and I must say hon, it brought the tears to my eyes to think you were about to go to the hospital and had no money. Did you use all the money that was in the bank? I thought you had got the separation money alright. You will have to go to a lawyer to see about it. I can't bear to see you want for anything hon and before I see you wanting I will sell anything and everything - the house too, if need be. I wrote Fred [his brother] a letter tonight that will open his eyes. I told him if my half of the gear wasn't worth anything to him that I would have it sold because I'm not going to see you want for anything. God knows hon I am bad enough off myself but I will live on one meal a day to help you. I can't bear it to think that you are bad off. I am going to write to father tonight and I will have it carried out about the sale of the nets if we can't come to an understanding some way.

Cal and I are out in the woods together writing letters and the both of us are pretty lonesome. Poor Cal feels pretty blue over the news he got. This is awful writing hon and you will have to excuse it because I am writing on top of my cap and it don't work very well. I hope you can make it out alright. I sent my boots to be repaired and all I have is a pair of P.T. shoes. I can't get uptown until I get my boots back. How are they all at home? I mean your home and your grandmother. I hope she is well. Is Tony home yet? Did you ever get any money from old Gardener? I wrote him a pretty stiff letter and I told father too about it. It wouldn't do hon to sell my half of the fishing gear you know because when I went back I wouldn't have any gear and you know he will keep it all in repair. Just the same I will see that you get your share dear. Well love, I think this will be all for this time so hoping you and the little fisherman are both well I will say bye, bye darling with a million kisses and all our love.

HARRY HECKBERT

I am forever your old man. Give Johnny a great big hug for me

Not every letter Harry receives from Iva cheers him up—she too experiences the blues. Harry has given up waiting for a telegram about the birth; he will wait for a letter. He now realizes that the money he received was his share of the fish money from his father and brothers. This, in turn, explains why Iva is broke. All this stress causes Harry to muse about the money he had spent in former years on rum. He assures Iva he has not behaved that way in England, if for no other reason than that he has not had the necessary funds. He promises that, upon his return, he will be a different man.

August 10, 1918
Bramshott Camp
My Dear Wife,

I got another letter from you today and I must say it cheered me more than the one I got last night. It was one of your bad days alright when you wrote that one and hon dear, it was one of my bad nights when I answered it. If I said anything out of the way you will have to excuse me as that note of Fred's got my goat. Dear I wouldn't like to tell you all I said in the letter I wrote to him. I certainly felt blue last night and it is no wonder to think I have so mean a brother. I had a letter from father today and he said it was him, Billie and Fred that sent me that money. Papa gave me 10 dollars and what Fred and Billie sent me, it must have come out of the fish or I wouldn't have got it. I am writing them tonight and telling them it would look better if they would think of you before me. If I had known how you were situated about money I would have sent it all to you dear as bad as I needed it. When I read your letter today, it certainly made me feel better dear because since last night I have been worrying about you.

If I just could get my hands on old Gardener for one minute I would be satisfied and I guess he would be too. I am glad hon they cut out the rum in Summerside because the old miser can't get any now. I never had a half dozen drinks of liquor since I came to England but I had some beer and not very much of that because I can't afford it. It certainly makes me think dear of all the money I wasted. Just think dear if I had one quarter of it now, how much it would help you out now, but it can't be helped now hon. Believe me, when I get back I will be a different man. The money they sent me is all gone now. I had to buy a suit, soap, towels and quite a lot of stuff and believe me they see a soldier coming and charge him two prices for everything. I don't like the thoughts of you renting a couple of rooms in town for the winter. Oh hon wouldn't it be much better to live in your little home than to do that? It would cost a lot for rent and you would have to have coal just the same. But I know how you feel hon, and you know you have my heartfelt sympathy but the way the war looks now it looks as if the Germans are on the run. I hope to God they are. I gave up looking for the telegram altogether now and will wait patiently for a letter. Well, sweetheart. cheer up because I feel it in my bones there is better days handy although I felt so rotten last night. Dearest, I guess, I will close for this time so good bye sweetheart.

Another Sunday with nothing to do but reflect on the minister's prayers for loved ones and feel lonesome. Add the effect of guilt over the "fish money," and Harry is one sad boy. The preacher again has warned the men about the temptations of the flesh, and Harry assures Iva once more of his immunity, for he is a family man. He lives in hope of better days to come, of the war's end, and of a letter from home announcing the birth of a son.

August 11, 1918
Bramshott Camp

My Dear Wife,

This is Sunday and a long lonesome day it is too. I guess I wrote you a letter nearly every day but here goes for another. I had a letter from Willie about an hour ago and he said the money Fred and him sent me was the fish money. If I had known that when I got it and the way you were situated I would have sent it back to you although hon I needed it very bad. And to think I had been writing to you for money and you had none for yourself, but hon I didn't know how everything was situated. You will have to excuse me. Well sweetheart, I expect everything is all over by this time. I have given up looking for a telegram but am anxiously waiting for the news. Oh hon I hope you are alright by this time. You don't know how I feel sometimes when I think how far away from you I am and you sick too. I will hope and pray that everything is alright. I was at church this morning and when the minister began to pray for all our loved ones at home a big lump came in my throat that nearly chocked me. Sunday is the worst day of all for me. Nothing to do but worry. I will be going back to my Reserve the last of next week and I expect they will drill the devil out of me, but if they work me too hard I will queer them again. If I wasn't married and like some of them here I would go to France tomorrow, but I don't want to go the way I am situated because one day I am coming home to my dear wife and kiddie and the less chances I take the better. I am going to send home a letter I got from Lena in this one. I haven't heard from her for a while. The preacher spoke about the young men's temptation, you know, he meant with women, but you know hon if they were all like me, there would be no need to tell them because I would no more think of anything of that then I would of committing suicide. I suppose Ethel is there by this time. You must tell her as she is out home that talk starts very easy there and to look out for it. Sweet, I guess I will have to say Bye for now.

Harry is so excited that he forgets to date his next letter. He has finally received the news: he is a father. Charles Lloyd Heckbert was born on July 18. It has taken about a month for Harry to receive the word. The news so cheered him that he forgot to "fall out" of his route march that day. He hopes mother and child, whom he dubs the "little fisherman," are both well. He relates plans to visit a family acquaintance on an upcoming leave, and assures Iva of his fiscal prudence while in England.

August ___, 1918
Bramshott Camp

Hello Sweetheart,

Congratulations. I received two letters from you today with the good news, "O.K." Oh sweetheart, how proud I am and how glad too that everything is alright. A little fisherman too, just think I told you what it would be, didn't I? He must be pretty if he looks like the old man (ha, ha). I am so glad he has got my good nature. Oh hon, you can't imagine how bug I feel now to be called daddy and you must give him a big kiss for me, won't you? I hope you isn't disappointed because it is a boy. You must get your pictures taken as soon as you can and send me one right off. You won't be so lonesome now or at least I hope you won't anyway, but I know dear you must be lonesome. I know I am. I found a four-leafed clover last night, the first I saw in England. I just said to myself, everything is alright and this is good luck and it came true sooner than I expected. The old man must have gotten quite a surprise when your mother told him. I know dear he will be good to you and the baby.

When I get my pay I will buy a little broach with baby sheep on it and send it home. I saw some the other day.

I was out on a long march today and I'm pretty tired now. I didn't fall out either, the good news cheered me up so much I forgot to fall out. I bet I will dream about him tonight. Some weight to him, I kind of thought he might be very small but if he weighed 8 pounds he is no toy. I hope you are well again by now and baby too, dear. I got a letter from Mr Newsham today and when I get my pass I am going down to his place. It is about 200 miles from here. It won't cost so much. When I get my pass, I am going to wire to old Gardener for money. I guess he will send it alright. Please don't think I am extravagant over here dear, but it takes a lot of money to get along and I don't waste it either. Oh hon, if I could just walk in tonight. What a meeting it would be. Well dear, I guess I will have to close for this time, so with two million kisses and all kinds of love I will say bye, bye dear.

Although Harry is now back with the Reserve Battalion and doing drill, all is fine, and in his next letter there is a notable absence of any mention of being lonely. He approves of the name Charles for their boy, but wonders where it came from. He has encountered yet another Island boy, this time from O'Leary—a fellow who knew Iva's family well. He gives Iva some financial advice, and tells of his plans to go to Manchester while on leave.

August 18, 1918
Bramshott Camp
My Dear Wife,

This is Sunday afternoon and I am back at my Reserve. I will be on parade in the morning. I am pretty well and hope that this will find you and Charles the same. Say hon, I think that name is alright. Did you hit on it yourself or did someone suggest it? I think it will be fine. I was in my class the other day and a little short fellow was next to me. I asked him where he was from and he said O'Leary. Then I asked him his name and he said Brooks. I said I bet you know my wife and when I told him who she was he said, for God sake, I guess, I do know her. He said he was related to Luther Crossman. We had quite a long talk. He came to the 17th Reserve the same day as I did, but I haven't seen him since as he is in a different company.

Oh hon, I hope you are both well. Did you get your separation money yet? You said you would have to take money out of the bank to pay the hospital bill. I thought you took that all out long ago to live on when you wasn't getting any. You say you will put it back when you get your separation but it will take all you get dear to live on and don't run short for the sake of putting it in the bank. I heard from Earl the other day. Do you know the girl he goes with? He sent me a snapshot with the letter—some Kite alright! Does Bruce still go with McDougall? I sent Bruce a book today that I got at the museum. I thought it would interest him.

I wired the old Gardener for some money to go on pass with. I am going to Manchester to see Mr and Mrs Newsham. I will be going in about two weeks time as far as I know. I don't know if he will send me the money or not, but if he don't I will go just the same as I get my carfare on the train for free and it won't cost me anything when I get there. I expect that letter I wrote him when I was mad will get his goat. I want you both to get your pictures taken as soon as you can and you know what to do with one, don't you? If you don't you will soon hear from me. I had a letter from Mr Newsham and they were tickled to death to think that I was going up. I have to go through London so you see I will see quite a lot.

Well sweetheart, I guess I will have to ring off once more so with two million kisses and all kinds of love, I am yours forever bye, bye sweetheart.

Harry experiences an unexpected setback. Transferred back to the Reserve Battalion, he was out on parade, and now he's scheduled for another Medical Board visit. Too stiff for drill, he tells Iva, although he also admits to having dirty equipment, too. Still, Harry doesn't seem too upset even if it does mean another indefinite delay in obtaining his leave. Oddly, he insists on calling his son "Johnny" even though he approved the moniker "Charles." His continuing this practice to describe his "little fisherman" makes one wonder if he truly approved of Iva's choice.

August 20, 1918
Bramshott Camp

My Dear Wife,

This is Tuesday afternoon and I came back to Reserve Battalion last Friday night. I went on parade one day and was put up for another Medical Board. I do not have to drill any until I get my board. They put me to work in the cookhouse and I beat it to write this letter. I got a letter from you at dinner time and was awful glad to hear that you and the baby are well. They don't know what to make of me here. I can't drill, my arms and legs are too stiff. Oh hon, how I would like to see little Johnny and give him a big kiss. You must get your pictures taken and send me one as soon as you can. There is no excuse now you know. I am up for office in the morning for having dirty equipment, but I don't mind that now, I am getting used to it. I don't know when I can go on my pass now on account of being up for Board but I will get it sometime. I suppose you are out home by this time. Well hon you will have to excuse this short letter this time. I will write tomorrow, so with tons of love for you. I will say bye, bye.

Harry is feeling down again because, although he lost his chance at leave, his chum Cal has gone to Scotland. Harry had even written his brother Fred for leave money, and now if it arrives he plans to bank it with the Salvation

Army. This is telling as to just how extensive were the services the Salvation Army provided the troops. Harry is so down that he is taking unwise risks. He relates just escaping an officer while on reduced cookhouse duty and of writing letters on the "Government's time." If he had been caught, he would have regretted his recklessness.

August 21, 1918
Bramshott Camp

My Dear Wife,

I received another letter from you last night and was awful glad hon to hear that you were both well. I am glad the baby is good. I guess he gets that from the old man. I certainly do feel lonesome here hon these days. To think that I am so far away from my sweetheart but as that piece on the gramophone used to say, "a million miles and far between us two." Cal Chappell is going on his pass today but I can't get mine now as I am up for Board. I am getting so now I don't care much whether I get it at all or not. I sent to Fred to get some money to go on pass with but that was before I was put up for Board. I am sorry now I sent for it but if he sends it I will put it in the Salvation Army Bank until I want it. Well sweetheart, news is scarce now as I very seldom go anywhere but I will write often although I haven't very much news. Well sweetheart, I guess I will have to close once more with a million kisses for yourself and another for our boy....

Well hon this is the 22nd I saw the officer coming yesterday and I had to beat it. I was writing on the Government's time but I saw him coming just the same. I am supposed to be working in the cookhouse now but I beat it to finish this letter. Cal Chappell went on his pass yesterday and went to Scotland. He had a sore back and can't drill very much. I really believe his back is sore. When I go on my pass I will try and get something

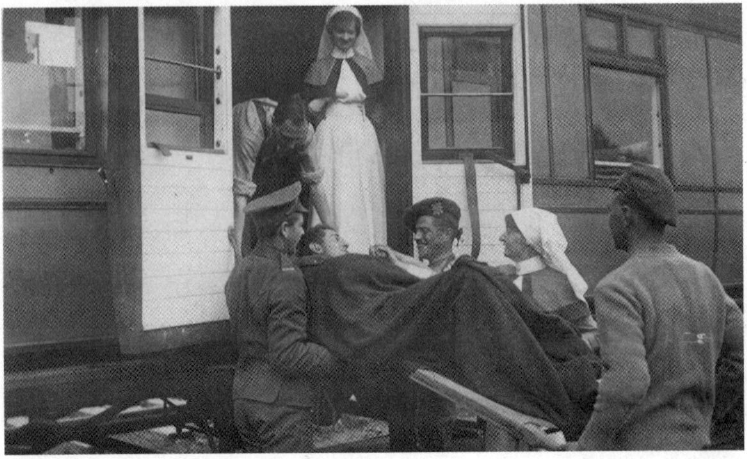

A soldier being loaded into a hospital train.

for the little girls and something for our little boy. Oh hon, I am awful proud of him. I wouldn't call the King my uncle now (ha, ha) I don't know what I will get out of the Medical Board this time but I expect to get "B." Anyway it will cost you a lot for coal and things and if you can't get enough to get along I will have to sell the nets because I can't see you wanting for anything dear. Well sweetheart I will close for this time, with millions of kisses to you and the baby.

Harry's Medical Board hearing took place on August 23. His file records that the medical officer determined "he cannot carry on as an 'A' category," so Harry became a "B1." Harry is anything but disappointed; as he relates to Iva, "no more drilling for this chicken" and the new designation "gave me a good job and lots to eat." Harry is back at the cookhouse and loving it. He tells of a great feed of "green beans and vinegar." The money has arrived from brother Fred, and he is now making plans to spend it when he goes on leave to visit the Newshams in Manchester.

August 29, 1918
Bramshott Camp

My Dear Wife,

This is Thursday afternoon and I have struck a new job. I am working in the sergeants' mess, some job! Roy Wadman[35] and I work together. I am all through soldiering! I had my Medical Board a few days ago and got marked "BI" so they gave me a good job and lots to eat. I thought I would get something out of them after a while. I got the money from Fred alright, but didn't go on pass yet. I will be going soon. I heard from Mr Newsham yesterday and they want me to let them know when I can go to see them. Well sweetheart, I hope you are both well. I am feeling fine now but I don't want to get too smart. I have to keep my eye peeled for something better, no more drilling for this chicken. I only had my rifle and equipment on the square one day and that got their goats and believe me it got mine too. Four doctors examined me. Believe me I gave them a stream of bull.

Oh hon, if I could only get back to see our dear baby but I am expecting a picture soon. Mr and Mrs Newsham wished us all kinds of congratulations and happiness imaginable. I heard last night that that Cody fellow who used to work in the station at Summerside died in the hospital here. I had a nice feed of green beans and vinegar for dinner today—some feed. I think I will get fat here (ha, ha)

I haven't got any letters for a week and every time I see the mail man I think sure he has some for me. How are they all home? Is Tony in Summerside now? How is your mother, grandmother and all the rest? I will try and get the little girls something when I go on pass. Did you get your separation money yet? I suppose whenever you get some money you will be buying a carriage for our little son. I suppose he won't hardly be big enough to work this winter, will he? Ha, ha. But it is surprising how fast

35 Roy Wadman (3204142), born at Central Bedeque, Prince Edward Island, 1883; conscripted in Charlottetown on February 25, 1918.

they grow up. All the boys here tell me how lucky I am. I said, "if you had a home and a wife would you think you were lucky to be thousands of miles away from them?" They don't look at it the way I feel. I will admit it was a lucky move for me when I got BI.

Well dear, I will close with love to little Johnny and his new mother; yours forever, you old man Hal.

Harry is a happy man. He is so upbeat that he writes Iva before he even mails his previous letter—both letters go in the same envelope. His new job is a "dandy," and going by his description not very demanding. He handles the dishes for the officers' mess, but he does not have to wash them himself!

August 30, 1918
Bramshott Camp

This is Friday and I am having a pretty good time. I have a dandy job. I eat with the sergeants too—some class A. I think I will be going on pass next week and I will try and get some little things for the kids. I wrote you a letter yesterday and had no envelope so I guess I will put this in the same envelope. I certainly am glad I got this job because I haven't hardly anything to do. I don't even wash a dish. All I have to do is to carry out the dishes to the wash house after they are done eating, then after they are washed I carry them back and set the tables again. With that it is all over till the next meal.

Well hon I haven't much news this time, so bye, bye dear with a million kisses for both of you, I remain yours forever, Harry

Still holding down his new job, Harry jots down a note telling of letters received and admits to having little new to tell. He does, however, mention in passing that he is sporting two new sets of teeth, and nice ones at that! The army did grant Harry some benefits after all. He does let one telling tidbit drop, though: he admits that he is envied by the other men for having gotten out of drill.

August 31, 1918
Bramshott Camp

Hello Sweetheart,

This is Saturday afternoon and I am holding the old job down yet. I got three letters this morning, but the one I was looking for didn't come. That was yours. I expect I will get some from you tomorrow. I had one from [sister] Flossie. What do you know about that and one from Jayne Halley and one from Earl. I got a new suit the other day. I tell you hon I am some sport now. Did I tell you before that I have two new sets of teeth and nice ones too? A lot of the boys are jealous of me here because I don't have to drill but I should worry they have the same chance I got but haven't got guts enough. I suppose you will think I have it pretty bad now writing nearly every day but hon I just can't help writing to you. Most every day I take a spell and think about home and everybody and everything then I just have to set down and write some kind of stuff. There isn't very much news, so I will close for now.

Harry continues in a good mood. He is still setting tables for the officers, but he rejoices that he has turned in his rifle and has no more brass to shine. There is even a rumour afoot that all B category men will be sent back to Canada. Harry is at this point unaware that, although the Canadians are making significant advances on the battlefield, these victories are coming at great cost. The Canadian Corps will suffer 30 percent of its casualties of the entire war in the final one hundred days. To sustain this effort, all men will be needed, and Harry will not be going home early.

September 4, 1918
Bramshott Camp

My Dear Wife,

This is Wednesday afternoon and I isn't working very hard these days. I am all through drilling. I am still in the Sergeants' Mess Room, some job! I had three letters from the Island lately but didn't get any from you for eight or ten days. I hope you isn't forgetting to write hon, but a fellow over here thinks all sorts of stuff. I can't tell what day I may be leaving here. I expect they will be putting me on some job or other. I would just as soon leave here as not. I don't think much of this place. I hear they are going to send a lot of B men back to Canada. I hope it will be my luck to be one of them. Well sweetheart, I suppose you are settled down out home again. Is Ethel out with you? Did you get the separation money yet? How is little Johnny getting along? I suppose he is growing. Did you get the carriage yet? I know there is not a lot of news in my letters dear, but I try and fill them with something and I know dear you like to get them too. Oh hon, you don't know the feeling that comes over me when I get one of your letters. How is the dear boy? I suppose he still has the good nature like his father, (ha, ha). I must try and write to Aunt Jemimah this afternoon. She said she was going to send me some socks soon. That will be fine. You ought to see me setting tables for the sergeants, nice white tablecloths and plates and cups, none made of old tin plates like I used to eat out of, some class. I haven't any rifle or equipment now. I turned all the stuff in and haven't any brass to shine now! Believe me I am not sorry either. Well sweetheart, you will be getting tired reading this old stuff, so I guess I will close for this time so with two million kisses and a ton of love for both of you I will say, bye, bye sweetheart.

Yours forever, your old man, Harry

The rumours persist and Harry is moved. He now finds himself at the Nova Scotia Regimental Depot, but not really any closer to a return to Canada.

September 7, 1918
Bramshott Camp

My Dear Wife,

This is Saturday and they have moved me again. I am at the N.S.R.D. now—that is the Nova Scotia Regimental Depot. They are all Category B men here, no drilling at all. I believe they will be sending me away somewhere on one job or another. I hear today that all Category B men are going home to Canada. Oh sweetheart, if that is only true and I can get home, won't it be great? There is a great lot of them here and they have to make room for the good men somehow. I only hope it is true.

Even though a lot of the men who came from Canada when he did are over in France, Harry clearly does not expect to go. He is lonesome and rather impatient. In response to a question from Iva, he assures her she is not running around too much, and he is confident of her fidelity. His brother Fred gives him a great surprise by sending him money and promising more if needed. The funds are in the Salvation Army Bank awaiting his leave.

September 8, 1918
Bramshott Camp

My Dear Wife,

This is Sunday afternoon and a lonesome old day for me and raining besides. I was to church this morning and it made me feel worse still when the minister started to pray for our loved ones at home. It started the tears when I thought of you and baby all alone at home, but cheer up dear because I really believe that better days are handier than we expect. All the same dear it gets my goat to think that they are keeping me here but I will get their goats once in a while anyway. A lot of the boys who came over when I did are in France now. I got your letter yesterday and believe me I was glad to hear that you are both well. No sweetheart, I don't think that you are running around too much because I know that you are true. You know hon you can depend on me to be true too. But don't go and give the neighbours things to talk about. You know I want you to enjoy yourself and you can and you just want to take it as easy as you can. I am taking it easy over here. Believe me they never will get any good out of me but I get so lonesome sometimes I don't know what to do. To think of them keeping me over here doing nothing.

Well dear, how is the boy getting along? I would just love to see him. I hope he is better looking than his daddy. I had a letter from father yesterday and he certainly praised our boy up so he must be alright. What do you think? I had a letter from Fred and he said anytime I wanted money he would send it to me. I never got such a surprise since I have been in the army as when I read that letter. I don't know whether I get all your letters or not. I only got one this last two weeks. I wrote quite a lot to you this last two weeks, of course, they wasn't very interesting letters but sweetheart it was the best I could do. There isn't very much news here that I can tell so I just have to fill the letters with all kinds of stuff. I didn't go on my pass yet because they have been moving me around so much.

I didn't have any chance to get a pass. I put the money that Fred sent me into the Salvation Army Bank till I go on pass so I wouldn't spend it. I haven't been out of camp for over three weeks. I don't care if I go anywhere or not. Dwight tells me I am getting too lazy to go anywhere. It is different with him. I suppose if I weren't married I would be running around too, but now no running around for me, I am through hon. Do you hear from Allan often? I wrote to him but didn't get any answer. The Canadians are certainly putting it on old Fritz now. I often think about Allan. Well sweetheart, I will have to close for his time and so hoping you and baby are well and happy.

Harry admits his previous letter wasn't very cheery, but Iva's next one cheered him up. Harry, in a very fatherly mood, suggests splitting with his son the ten cents Iva plans to send him for a celebratory beer. Iva still hasn't received any separation allowance from the government, and Harry is gaining weight.

September 9, 1918
Bramshott Camp

My Dear Wife,

I wrote you a letter yesterday when I was feeling kind of blue as I always do on a Sunday. I might have said something that would make you feel bad but hon I hasten to excuse myself. I had a letter from you last night and was awful glad to hear that you and baby are well. I am glad he is a good boy, that's what it is to have a good father (ha, ha) and about that ten cents you are going to send me to buy beer. I don't think you should. Wouldn't it be better to give half to our boy to blow himself with and I have no objection to taking the other half. Hon, what do you think? I am glad you got a good carriage when you were about it. It is the cheapest in the end. Oh sweetheart, if I could only see our boy. I am glad your grandmother likes him. I guess the old man likes him too by the way he spoke of him in his letter. He must be some boy alright. I am surprised to think you didn't get your money yet. There must be something the matter with the whole business. I am going to see if I can do anything here about it. Poor Tom Clark, he must feel bad when he can't get his booze. It is a long while since I had a drink of liquor. Any time I feel as I can afford it I have a drink of beer. One glass of this beer is as good as a dozen of that stuff they used to sell there. I got weighed the other day and I weigh 182 pounds. I am getting fat! Well hon I guess I will close for this time so with love and kisses to you

Harry has news: he is being moved. What all this will entail and portend for his future remains to be seen, but for the time being he is unconcerned.

September 11, 1918
Bramshott Camp

My Dear Wife,

I am leaving Bramshott tomorrow for Shorncliffe. I don't know what kind of a job they got for me but it better be a pretty easy one. I wrote you a letter yesterday and haven't much news . Will write whenever I get settled.

Well sweetheart, bye, bye once more.Harry

Harry learns that Iva has received the separation allowance money, and just in time, too. Harry was intending that very day to march into the colonel's office and demand to know what was the matter! Iva's good news is also accompanied with the promised ten cents for a celebratory beer. Harry enjoyed his first and then, despite his earlier thoughts of sending the other five cents home to his boy, became very thirsty and had another. He's sure Iva will understand. After all, she now has the funds to give the little fisherman five cents any time she wishes.

September 11, 1918
Bramshott Camp

My Dear Wife,

I wrote you a few lines this morning and just after mailing it I got a letter from you. Believe me dear, I was awful glad to hear you got your separation money because I was going to parade before the Colonel this afternoon to see about it and that is a job I don't like much. You will be able to pay your bills now sweetheart but you will find it costs so much to live now that you won't be able to put any away. Thanks very much honey for that ten cents. I had a pint of beer on the head of it. I was going to send half of it back for our boy to blow himself with but really I was thirsty and I thought perhaps you wouldn't mind giving him five cents, you are so rich now ha, ha.

I don't remember what I done with my cufflinks honey, I always thought I left them in my shirt but some dirty bugger might have stole them in Charlottetown. It is too bad because you know how I prized them. I am glad you heard from Mrs Allen and the rest of them asking you up to their place and I am glad you went too. Some class to the old man. I near dropped dead when I read the letter. Is that the Mrs Mountain that used to live by Mrs Burns's? I will have to go through London tomorrow on my way to Shorncliffe so I suppose I will see some sights.

I got a letter from uncle Charlie today and he said he saw my loving wife when he was down. If he just knew how I love her though he would say more than that. He said if I wanted any money just let him know. You know dear I wouldn't ask him for money although I know I would get it quick. I am going to write to him this afternoon. Well sweetheart, this is the second letter I wrote you today. You will say I have it pretty bad now and dear I guess I have too, but never mind dear I am looking forward to the time when I will be going home. Then oh hon what a big hug and kiss, first thing. Well sweetheart, I have lots of paper today. I suppose about two dozen sheets and envelopes to take with me so I won't run short for a while. I will use some whenever I land in my new place. I guess I will close again, so try and be happy until your old man returns, then everything well be alright. Love to you and baby.

Harry even has bigger news: not only has he been moved to Shorncliffe Camp, but it appears they intend to send him to France as part of a work battalion.

September 12, 1918
Shorncliffe Camp

My Dear Wife,

I have arrived in Shorncliffe O.K., but sweetheart, I think they are going to send me to France in a working Battalion. Don't be discouraged dear because I isn't going to walk very far for them and a man that can't walk is no good there. I haven't got time to write much now but will write later.

Piles of love and kisses from your old man, Harry

Harry is not happy, but he is resigned to going to France unless he can "queer them" at another Medical Board hearing. He tries to comfort and cheer Iva despite the news. He knows no one at this camp. He tells her that he will write faithfully, although the mail will not keep up to him, so the conversation will be very lopsided.

September 15, 1918
Reinforcement Company General Depot, Shorncliffe

My Dear Wife,

This is Sunday afternoon and I am in Shorncliffe. I don't like the place very well. I think they are going to send all "BI" men to France. Well sweetheart, I suppose I have as much right to go as the rest. The only reason I have for not going dear is for you and baby's sake. I know it will make you feel bad and Lord knows you must feel bad enough now, but don't get discouraged dear. Everything will be alright in the end. They won't give me my pass at all now. They are all cancelled. I waited a little too long. I don't care much for that as I wouldn't enjoy it very much anyway. I am going to make them give me another Board before I go to France and I might queer them yet. I haven't any idea when I will be going but will write as often as I can. I don't feel bad about it hon, only for your sake so try and keep up your courage and all will be well. I was to the Church of England this morning and when I came from there I went to the Salvation Army and am here writing. I don't know when I will get any letters now. You know dear when a fellow moves it takes two or three weeks to get your mail and very often you don't get it at all. I will be looking for some from you all the time. There isn't one soul I know here and you can imagine how lonesome I am. God knows it was bad enough before but it is nothing to worry dear, the war won't last very much longer anyway. We will have to look on the bright side of life just now. Well dear, I don't feel like writing any more now so I guess I will have to close.

Harry's isolation continues, and his hut mates are not his favourite people. Harry, representative of his day, is a long way from embracing linguistic diversity.

September 17, 1918
Shorncliffe Camp

Dearest Wife,

Just a line to tell you I think I am booked for France. Don't be discouraged dear because I ain't sure yet if I am going or not. I hope you and baby are well dear. I am feeling pretty blue these days, not a single soul I know here and I am in a hut where there is a lot of Quebec French and the way they chew the rag nearly sets me crazy. Well dear, you will have to excuse this short letter as I don't feel like writing much but will try and do better next time. So I will say bye, bye dearest.

Harry is now on the English coast, near Dover, and he can see the flashes of the artillery in France at night. He says it "looks awful." Although he hasn't been through the gas or musketry tests yet, Harry still feels he might be sent to France. He relates a very interesting incident to Iva about an encounter in town with two girls in uniform who took pity on a lonely Canadian. If Harry looked as lonesome as he sometimes sounded, it is no wonder the two girls, in all innocence, kindly stopped to chat.

September 18, 1918
Reinforcement Coy General Depot
Shorncliffe

Dear Wife,

This is Wednesday afternoon and I am not doing anything yet. I don't know for sure if I am going to France or not as all the rest of the boys that came here with me are passing their gas test and musketry and I never done anything yet. So I can't tell yet. I never had a letter from you for a long while. I know you write them dear but the mail gets all mixed up when a fellow moves. How are you and baby sweetheart? I hope you are both well. I am pretty well but awful lonesome sometimes. I was in town on Sunday and oh Hon what a lovely place it is. There is a dandy beach and lots of seats. I was wandering all alone when two girls dressed in khaki said to me "hello Canada." I said hello when one of them said "you look lonesome." I said, "believe me I am." One said sit down on the beach for a while. I said no girls I can't because I am a married and I respect my wife too much for that. She said, you mistake us, we isn't the kind that you think we are. We thought you were lonesome and that's why we stopped. I bade them goodbye and left. They might have been good girls alright but Hon I couldn't walk with a girl, no sweetheart. I love you and respect you too much for that. We are handy to France here and can see it on a clear day and see the sky lit up by night, it looks awful. I hope you are getting along alright. How is everybody down home? I would love to see them all. Well, I will close once more.

Harry writes again but with little news. He tells Iva there is noise in his hut—"too much chewing going on"—and that he remains without both letters or any clear sense of his immediate future.

September 19, 1918
Reinforcement Coy General Depot, Shorncliffe

My Dear Wife,

Just a line to let you know I am still on the map yet. I wrote you a line yesterday but the paper wasn't any good and there was too much chewing for me to write much. I have been in this place a week today and haven't done anything yet and don't know what I will be doing yet. All the boys who came here with me are passing their gas test and musketry but I haven't been called out of the hut yet. I can't tell for sure yet if I will have to go to France or not. I never had a letter from you for a long while. I know you write them dear but a lot of them goes astray every time they move me. Well dear, how are you and baby getting along? I hope alright but I know you must find it hard alone. I hope you isn't as lonesome as I am sometimes. There is a nice town handy the camp here but I very seldom go down. I don't feel like going anywhere. I am glad you got your money alright for you must need it. I guess I will close.

The sobering casualty news from the great Canadian advance has reached Harry. He has heard that a lot of Island boys have been killed. He worries about Allan and his chum Cal. The reality of war, even when your side is winning, occupies Harry's thoughts.

September 21, 1918
Reinforcement Coy General Depot, Shorncliffe

My Dear Wife,

This is Saturday afternoon and I thought I would write you a few lines to let you know I am still here. I haven't done anything since I came here. I don't know yet what they are going to do with me. I hear that there is a lot of boys killed from the Island. I would like to know their names. Do you ever hear from Allan? I wrote to him when you sent me his address and never heard from him yet. I often wonder dear how he is getting along. I guess I wrote you five or six letters this week .Surely you will get some of them. I never got any letters since I came here, not even from the boys at

Bramshott. I wrote Cal Chappell whenever I landed here. I expect I will be getting a whole bag full of letters one of these days. Well dear, how are you and baby feeling these days? I hope you are both well. I suppose the baby is growing like a weed. Oh hon wouldn't I just love to see you and him. You must get a hustle on and get those pictures taken and send me one. I guess this will be all for this time.

Harry is dreaming about home, Iva, and the baby. He relates an interesting account of the soldiers' attitude toward the Salvation Army's presence in the camps. He says that, although the men patronize the huts for letter writing and food, they are much less likely to attend the religious meetings. Harry notes that he is an exception to this rule. One might conjecture that Harry found solace in the "meetings" and an understanding ear in the volunteer workers.

September 22, 1918
Reinforcement Coy General Depot, Shorncliffe
My Dear Wife,

This is Sunday afternoon and raining to beat the band. I wrote you yesterday but somehow or other I had to write again today. Well sweetheart, I dreamed I was home last night and oh hon, what a big hug you gave me. They can't be going to send me to France with the rest of the boys because they all got their packs today and I didn't get any.

I didn't go to church this morning because I was mess orderly and didn't get my dishes washed in time but I am going to the Salvation Army tonight. I was there Friday night when there was only six of us men there. As a rule the soldiers don't go to their meetings much, but they are glad enough to get in to write and get lunches. I would love to hear from you soon. It seems so long since I had a letter but I will just have to wait I suppose. I saw the baby just as plain as day in my dream last night and have been wondering ever since if it looked like him. I guess I will have to close for this time.

Harry wonders if the authorities have lost his name—he does not appear to be slated for any task, and he is not asked to do anything. As long as his name is not lost from the pay list, he is not too concerned!

September 24, 1918
Reinforcement Coy General Depot, Shorncliffe

My Dear Wife,

Here it is the twenty fourth of the month and I never got a letter since I came here. Oh hon, I am awful lonesome tonight. Most all the boys have gone up town but I don't care very much whether I go anywhere or not. I am not working at all. I think they must have lost my name altogether. I hope they did. Only for pay day, if my name wasn't on the list I wouldn't get any money. It is awful queer they haven't got me into something but believe me as long as they leave me alone I ain't going to look for a job. ha, ha. I fail to see where they are going to get their money's worth out of me. Don't you dear? I dreamed last night again I was home and I had two more fellows with me. I don't know who they were and we were sitting at the table in the kitchen eating.

Harry has big news: they have changed his categorization and he is back to soldiering! He is back at Bramshott Camp drilling in preparation for going to France. He tells Iva he is ready to go and do his bit. His only regret is that she is likely to worry too much, but Harry is confident the war will soon end. Also a source of cheer is that he has received his first letter from Iva in weeks. And it included snaps of her and the little fisherman. Harry is a contented soldier.

October 4, 1918
Bramshott Camp

My Dear Wife,

I received your letter last night and snaps too. Say hon, they were great. I am back to Bramshott drilling again. They raised my category at Shorncliffe so I am soldering again, but don't know how long it will last. I think the war is nearly over anyway so don't worry if I go to France dear. Be patient for a while yet and everything will be alright. I have a chance to get my leave but the money is all gone now. Dwight and Earl are about ready for France now. I intended to write before but hadn't enough time. I beat it off parade this afternoon to write this. Oh hon I would love to see the baby, he looks so nice. Joe Gillis went to France last night and Percy Dunsford[36] too. My hand shakes awful this afternoon, I take spells like that quite often and you will have to excuse this scribbling. I think I will try and drill now and go to France. The only thing that keeps me back is that I think you would worry if I went. If you will tell me you don't I will try to go and do my bit. Oh Hon I know you wouldn't like the idea. There must be something good in that boy where it cost that much and my mouth

36 Percy Dunsford (3204271), born in South Melville, Prince Edward Island, and living at Summerside, when conscripted in April 1918.

will be watering till I get it. I hope you and baby are well sweetheart and getting along alright. I have quite a bad cold now. We only get three blankets to sleep on and sleep right on the ground.

Are you thinking of going out home for the winter or staying down home? If you are going to stay home, what do you think of renting the house to someone? Mind I isn't telling you to rent it dear but if you like, you can. Use your own judgement. You would pick up a few cents that way but just please yourself about that dear. I bought a leather card case to put the snaps in so they wouldn't get broke. I bet you know which one I have in the front. I had it out about a dozen times today already looking at it. I showed them to Joe Gillis last night and he looked at each one about ten minutes. You ought to try and get some taken on post cards hon and send me one of each. That is the first letter I got since I came from Shorncliffe and believe me I was glad to get it, dear. I wrote to Fred to make arrangements for fishing and if the answer isn't satisfactory I will go about it a different way, but I think dear he will fix matters right. The last letter I had from him was pretty good. I got quite a surprise when he said he would send me some money any time I wanted it. Now sweetheart please don't worry about me for I will be alright and if I go to France I will crack a few Huns for you.

Guess I will close dearest, bye, bye

Harry has received a disagreeable letter from his younger brother Earl. Its contents are not revealed, but he sends it home to Iva and tells her not to say anything about it. It could well have contained some critical comments on Harry's fiscal relations with the folks at home while he was in uniform. We can safely assume that matters were subsequently smoothed over, for the letter in question is no longer extant.

October 6, 1918
Bramshott Camp

My Dear Wife,

This is Sunday and we are all quarantined in here. I got three letters from you yesterday. They had been on the way a long while and went to Shorncliffe before I got them. Well honey, I had a letter from our Earl and I am sending it to you. Please don't show it to anyone and don't tell anyone and please don't say anything about them or call them anything. I can't say I was very much pleased to get such a letter from Earl, but I suppose he wrote just what he thought. Guess this is all for now, will write tomorrow, love from Harry.

Again there is significant news: not only is Harry soldiering, but he is beginning to "like drill." He is ready to go to France. For the time being, however, no one is going anywhere, for the camp is quarantined. He cannot elaborate, but it is undoubtedly the "Spanish influenza" which struck in the autumn of 1918 and is ravaging all the armies on the continent. In the next few years, it will kill fifty thousand young Canadians on the home front. Moreover, the big news from home is related to Harry's father changing the family's fishing arrangements. The specifics are absent, but Harry thinks it means the other, younger sons, like Earl, will have to fend for themselves. Harry even thinks some of them will pack up and leave.

October 12, 1918
Bramshott Camp

My Dear Wife,

I received the box the other day and I tell you it came in a good time as I was hungry and broke. Besides, I also received three letters. Glad you and baby are well. I suppose you had a nice time in Shediac. I didn't know you were there until I got a letter from you saying you were over there. Yet I don't get half your letters and I don't suppose you get half of mine. I have been on the square two weeks drilling and really hon I am beginning to like it. If I can stand it I think I will go right through this time. I am getting tired of this place. I hope you won't worry dear because I will be alright. I must write to little Earl and put it in this letter. Well hon, I am surprised at the old man alright. I am sure it will make a change out home. I expect all the boys will beat it now. It would be a good thing if they had to get out and fish for themselves. They are old enough now to look after themselves. I had a letter from father yesterday and he never mentioned anything about it. I am surprised at myself now for liking drilling but really dear I am beginning to like it. I believe they will make a soldier of me yet. I got the papers and was awful glad to read the old Summerside news. Anytime you can send any more I will be awful glad to get them. We are all quarantined here and can't get out anywhere. I wish I could tell you more about it but I can't dear. I had a letter from Earl a few days ago and he told me about the old man. I bet Betsy will beat it to Boston now, won't she? Tell Fred Muttart and Ella I think they are real mean for not writing to me. I never got a scratch from either of them since I came here and I wrote to them several times. I hope everyone home is well and happy.

Well sweetheart, I guess I will say bye, bye Harry.

HARRY HECKBERT

Harry jots down a quick note telling Iva something he had forgotten to say in his previous letter.

October 13, 1918
Bramshott Camp

Hello Dear Wife,

I wrote you a letter last night and there was something that I forgot to say. If I go to France don't let the insurance agent know it or he will soak you when the time comes to pay up. You know if I went to France the insurance will cost a lot more and be sure and don't let him know. Guess I will ring off so, bye, bye.

Harry's soldiering has become much more serious. He is handling live bombs—actually, Mills bombs, an early form of grenade. Perhaps equally unhealthy, if he keeps it up, Harry has taken up smoking. He has smoked all the cigs Iva sent, and wonders how in the world she knew he had started smoking! Tellingly, he links his smoking to the flu pandemic, which he had heard erroneously helps keep the germs away. The flu is killing men before they even reach France.

October 16, 1918
Bramshott Camp

My Dear Wife,

This is Wednesday night and I thought it was about time to write my dear another letter. The weather is awful wet here. It rains every day. I am feeling pretty good these days and drilling every day. I was throwing live bombs this afternoon. I liked it fine and some of the boys were pretty nervous. Well sweetheart, I hope you and baby are getting along alright and are both well. Who did you send the cigarettes to dear? Was it to me? How did you know I learned to smoke? I smoked them all hon. They say it helps to keep germs away and I smoke one once in awhile but when I get out of this place I will cut it out.

I am beginning to like soldiering now and am getting along fine and don't be scared if I go to France because I will be alright. You wouldn't like for me to frig around here till the war is over, would you dear? When I went home they would say he went just as far as England. I am going right through darling so don't be scared. Hon, if I go over to France don't tell the insurance agent as I think you will have to pay a lot more insurance. I am going to get some pictures taken some time before I go over and will send them home.

I just came from tin town and I bought two shillings worth of cakes and my belly is pretty full now as I eat them all. What do you think about renting the house this winter? You know how if you don't want to, don't do it. Just use your own judgement. How are they all home? I hope they are all well and I suppose Tony is away about all the time. I hope your grandmother and mother and all the rest are well and happy. I am more contented here now because I like the drill so don't worry honey about me. Joe Wedge[37] and Ben Sonier[38] are here. I had a letter from Tommy Linkletter[39] from France and he likes the place pretty good. I never heard from Allen yet. Dwight got a letter from home the other day saying his brother was killed in France. He feels pretty bad about it. He is already for France but can't go until the quarantine is lifted. Well sweetheart I will have to close again, so bye, bye

Harry has received an old letter from Iva, one she penned a month ago.

37 Joseph Wedge (3204411), born Palmer Road, Prince Edward Island; conscripted May 1918 while living in Summerside.
38 Benjamin Sonier (3204631), born in Summerside, and conscripted from there in May 1918.
39 Thomas Linkletter (3204158), born in Summerside, and conscripted from there in March 1918.

Apparently he had received others more quickly. Under normal circumstances, the mail service was clearly doing quite well. The camp was still under quarantine. He tells of a feed of cakes shared with his chum, asks for a few cents' advance Christmas money, and tells of seeing an old flame of Iva's—one Percy Landrigan[40] of Kensington, Prince Edward Island, who was then in the Signals Corps.

October 17, 1918
Bramshott Camp

My Dear Wife,

This is Thursday evening and I got through my work early so I thought I would write my honey a few lines. I wrote last night but I have been thinking about you and baby all day so I just had to write again. I have been drilling all day and feel fine tonight . How I would love to walk into your home tonight and see you all. Oh, hon, what a squeeze you would get, but never mind. How I will be there some time perhaps sooner than we expect. I received a letter from you today but it was an old one dated Sept. 16 that was before you went to Shediac. I don't know where it has been all the time. I often get them that way. Who do you think I saw today? Percy Landrigan, that fellow Lee and you used to chase down at the station. Do you mind how it got your goat one night when I said you were chasing him (ha, ha) Tell Lee he looks fine and is on the signalling Corps. Did you hear from Allan lately? I hope he is all right. When are you going to send me a good picture of yourself and our dear baby. I hope it will be soon and are you going to send your old

40 Percy Landrigan (3204051), born in Kensington, Prince Edward Island, and conscripted for service in early 1918.

man a few cents for Christmas? You might think dear that I am hard on money over here. Well I guess I am but hon it all goes in my belly. Just the same. We can't get a drink of beer here now so the money lasts longer,

I wrote to your mother the other night and I hope she will get it alright. The time seems to go awful fast here now and I ain't sorry. It can't go too fast for me. I am longing for the day to come when I can get home to my dear wife and baby. Well hon, I guess I will try and finish this letter. A friend of mine just came in with a bag of cakes and asked me to have a lunch. He buys a bag one night and I buy one the next and we both set together so I feel a lot better now dear as my belly is full. You know I never feel good until I get a full belly. Well sweetheart, I guess I will close for this time, so hoping you and baby are well I will say bye, bye.

Harry is still at the base and still drilling, but the quarantine must have been lifted, for two of his friends have been hastily shipped to France. Harry expects to go fairly soon. He continues to train in preparation for leaving, including gas drill and shooting. He is concerned that Iva will worry too much, but on the positive side he tells her about his improved memory now that he is off the beer. He thinks he'll continue to abstain for the duration of his training.

October 19, 1918
Bramshott Camp

My Dear Wife,

This is Saturday night and I am well and still at the old camp. I am getting along pretty good drilling. I went through my gas test today, some stuff hon, one whiff of it will kill a man but we have good masks for protection. I expect in five or six more weeks hon I will be heading for France. I hope you won't worry about me dear. Just think of the old song, "what's the use of worrying, pack up your troubles in your old kit-bag and smile, smile, smile." I know it is hard for you dear to think of me going to France, but hon I know you will like for me to do my share, wouldn't you. Believe me when I get there, I will try my best to do it too. Now hon please don't worry about me, will you? You know I wouldn't want you to and it would make it harder for me if I knew you were worrying all the time. How is our dear boy? I hope you are both well. I would love to get some good pictures of you both before I go over. I don't think the war will last much longer anyway. Earl Reeves[41] and Philip Craig and some of my chums left here this evening en route to France. Earl hadn't time to write home to tell his mother so I promised him I would write her and tell her. I was shooting yesterday afternoon and made good too. I soon will be some soldier. I never had a drink of beer or anything for three weeks and hon I find that I can remember everything better than I could when I was taking some beer. You know hon what a poor memory I used to have. I believe that was partly the reason because I can remember all the things they tell me here. Believe me, we have something to remember. So I guess I will leave the beer alone till I get through training. Oh hon, if I just could think that you wouldn't worry too much it would make it easier for me. How is everyone at home? I hope they are well. I suppose Tony is away all the time. Will you be taking the base burner in home this winter? I think it would be great for you all in there and it wouldn't cost much more than the other one but you know best dear what to do yourself. I saw a book called "Canada Weekly" we get them here and there were quite a lot of Island boys names in the casualty list. I saw Arthur Gallant's[42] name from Summerside, would that be Mooney Po's? Well sweetheart, I guess I will have to close for now. So hoping you and baby are both well, also all the rest, I will say bye, bye.

41 Earl Reeves (3180368), born in Summerside and conscripted in February 1918 while living in Truro, Nova Scotia.

42 Arthur Gallant (712747), born 1897 at Howland, Prince Edward Island, son of Octave and Susan Gallant, killed in action, September 28, 1918.

Despite being broke again, Harry is in the best of spirits. He expects to go to France any day, but he is confident the war is almost over. He has been attached to The Royal Canadian Regiment, after almost having been placed in the 85th Battalion, a kilted Nova Scotia battalion first blooded at Vimy Ridge. Harry does not think he would have looked good in a kilt or enjoyed wearing one in winter weather. He hopes the folks at home are spared the flu. He has seen its work, and assures Iva that "it's awful."

November 10, 1918
Bramshott Camp

My Dear Wife,

This is Sunday and it is pretty cool here now. I expect to be going to France about Wednesday but don't expect to do any fighting as the war is just about over and I won't be there long. Cheer up hon for there are better days coming soon. I am feeling fine and hope you and baby are the same. Well sweetheart, everyone around here is in the best of spirits as there was some interesting news in the paper this morning. I have a bundle of badges to send home as we get already to leave. If they pay us before we leave I will send them before we go. I am broke now and can't send them home until I get some money. I never heard from you for about two weeks and am feeling anxious about you all for I heard the flu was raging there. I do hope to God hon that none of you will take it for it is awful. I am answering the defaulters call these days. I got three days CB [confined to barracks] for having a dirty rifle. I expected to get a few cents from you before I went to France but I have given up now. You said in one of your letters that you would send me some when you got your next cheque. But I suppose when you got it I was in Shorncliffe and you didn't know how long I would be there. Never mind dear, I got through without it although I went to bed pretty hungry sometimes. I am getting used to that now and don't mind it much. Do you ever hear from Allan? He never answered my letters and I can't help thinking about him. I am in the same Battalion as he is. The good old R.C.R. They pretty near had me in the 85th. Wouldn't I look funny in kilts, no chance of them getting kilts on me. They are a little too cool. Well sweetheart, I believe the war is just about over at last and it won't be long before I will be giving my darling a big hug as they will let the married men go first. I am on draft now and don't do any more parades (only the CB ha, ha) We might never go to France at all yet I would like to go over before I went home to see what it is like. I hope I will get some mail soon as I watch the mailman all the time. Well sweetheart, I guess I will have to close. Here's hoping you are all well and happy, I will say bye, bye

The war is over! Now there are flags and guards everywhere. There was quite a celebration and a good deal of vandalism channelled in one very particular direction: tin town, where the English merchants had set up shop just off the base to cater to the troops' needs. The soldiers smashed in, stole everything, and then burnt the remains. Serves them right, says Harry, they had fleeced everyone. Ironically, he hopes to get down there so he can mail a bundle of souvenir badges home to Iva. Such is the love/need/hate relationship that exists between tin town and the troops.

November 14, 1918
Bramshott Camp

My Dear wife,

I received your letter last night and was more than glad to hear from you because it was nearly three weeks since I got your last letter. Well hon, times have changed around here these last few days. We are on draft for France but I don't think they will send us over there. There are all kinds of yarns going around here. They certainly celebrated the victory here. They put tin town on the bum, broke all the stores down and swiped all the stuff. It served them right because they certainly were a gang of robbers. The place is under armed guards now. Everywhere one goes here he sees strings of flags flying. We isn't drilling any now, just lying around the huts. The Germans must have heard that I was going over and took cold feet. (ha, ha). I have a package of badges and if I can get over to tin town I will send them home today. I heard they are going to send us all to Canada, but that seems too good to be true. Never mind, hon, it won't be very long before I will be back again. I am awful glad you are all well. I never felt better in my life than I do now, the rheumatism don't bother me very much at all. We have our new badges now. They are dandy's, a big silver star with a gold crown in the centre. If I can swipe one anywhere I will send it home. I can buy one, but money is so scarce. We got paid yesterday and I had a can of sardines and a bottle of marmalade for breakfast this morning. I hope they won't keep me here in Bramshott all winter. I either want to go to Canada or France. Well hon, I guess this will be all for now, so bye, bye

Harry finally crosses the Channel, and lists his location as "Somewhere in France." He thinks the trip well worth it, for France is not such a bad place after all, excepting the mud, of course. They are constantly on the hike, so he doesn't expect any mail to catch up to him. He will nonetheless write faithfully. His thoughts turn to the approaching Christmas season. He has again dreamt of Iva, home, and the baby. He attended a moving picture show, and has seen many German prisoners, some of them very young, doing work under the watchful eye of guards.

November 21, 1918
Somewhere in France

My Dear Wife,

This is Thursday night and I got over at last. This isn't a bad country at all, only it is very muddy. I am well and hope this will find you and baby the same. We are on the hike now and when we get settled down I will write you. I suppose it will be months before I get any letters. Well dear, Christmas will soon be here won't it? We don't know how long we will be here, not very long I guess. I tell you hon this trip is worth something to a man. I only saw one man I knew since I came here and that was Gordon Arbing.[43] It is pretty cold at nights here but we don't mind it much. They feed us better here than they did in England. I can't give you any address now because we are pulling out of here in a few days and we don't know where we are going. I hope you will get my letters alright. I don't expect to get any for a long while now. If we go up to join our Battalion I might see Allan if he is there as I belong to the same Battalion. I dreamed I was home last night and I thought our boy could talk. I could see him so plain. I thought he had an awful lot of freckles. How is the old man getting along with his mountain. I hope alright. Never mind hon, your old man will soon be home once more. It will be like starting all over again won't it? Dear when I get up the line I must try and get some good souvenirs. How is Tony? Is he home now? I suppose men are very scarce there now. I went to a moving picture show the other night. The first one I was to since I left old P.E.I. The pictures were great. The soldiers go in free. We struck here Saturday for shorter hours and got them too. There is lots of German prisoners around here working with guards over them. Some of them just young fellows too.

43 Gordon W. Arbing (111014), born 1885 at Bedeque, Prince Edward Island, and residing in Summerside when he joined up in April 1915.

Well dear, I guess I will close, so wishing you and baby and all the rest at home and a very merry Christmas and Happy New Year.

I will say bye, bye with tons of love, your old man Hal Pte H. H. 3204333 RCR Batt France

Almost two weeks elapse before Harry's next letter. This one is unusual, for it is on Catholic Army Hut stationery instead of the typical YMCA letterhead. He was correct earlier—still no letters from home, although he expects a large instalment to arrive one day. He doesn't complain, for work is light and the food is good.

December 2, 1918
Canadian Corps Infantry School, France

My Dear Wife,

Just a line dear to give you my address. I heard we are going to be here for some time so I am sending my address so you can write. Well sweetheart, I am having a good easy time here. They feed us great so I have nothing to complain of only I would love to get home to my dear wife and baby, but the time will soon slip away dear. I don't know dear when I will get a letter from you. I know you write dear, there must be an awful pile somewhere. I expect to get a whole wheel barrow load some of these days. How are you all at home? I hope you are all well and happy. Did the insurance cost any more on account of me being over here. It shouldn't because the war was over before I got here. Well sweetheart, I guess I will have to close wishing you all a Merry Christmas and a happy new year I will say bye, bye.

A week passes, and Harry writes again on the usual YMCA stationary. No mail, no parcels, but life is good, for parade is only three hours a day and the food is great. He wishes he had a camera, for he was seeing some unusual sights, including grain coming up before Christmas. He wishes all at home a Merry Christmas.

December 9, 1918
France

My Dear Wife,

Just a line to let you know that I am well and having a good time. I never had any mail since I came here and don't know when I will get any. Well dear, Christmas is getting handy. I don't know if I will get any Christmas parcels or not. I hope I do. I would love to get a letter from you. I hope you are all well and happy. It won't be very long dear before your old man will be coming home. They feed us great here. We are only on parade three hours a day so we have a lot of time to ourselves but I very seldom go anywhere. There is so much mud. I suppose there is snow and ice down there by this time. The weather here is nice and warm, the grain is just coming up, it seems so funny to see grain coming up so handy to Christmas. I wish I had a camera, I would certainly get some funny snaps. I never saw anyone I knew over here but one. Where is Allan? Do you hear from him? I have been inquiring about him with the old soldiers but they don't know him.

Well dear, guess I will close, Wishing you all a merry Christmas and a happy New Year.

1919

Over a month passes before Harry's next letter. It is now 1919. Harry is again before the Medical Board, as is everyone else, and he is correct in assuming that this exam is to have implications for future pensions. Sadly, many troops who had been exposed to gas lied about how they felt at the time, fearing that if they admitted to a disability it would delay their discharge. This would have a serious effect on their future pension claims and those of their widows. Harry, fortunately, is spared this trouble. In other news, he has finally seen the Allan he has been asking after. He tells Iva he hopes to be home as soon as next month.

January 12, 1919

This is Sunday and I have just been up for a Medical Board. Everyone was up for one before we demobilize. I think it is about pensions.
Well sweetheart, we all expect to be home pretty soon. There is a rumour here that we will be aboard ship early next month. I believe it is true for they are fixing everything up. I saw Allan yesterday. He just got back off pass and had a good time. I am in an old stable writing this letter and it is pretty dark so you will have to excuse this writing. I hope to be home next month and we will be happy once more won't we dear? I am still in Belgium but we expect to move down shortly. Do you think you will be able to have our little home ready when I get back? If the stoves are in home I suppose you won't, but never mind dear. We will soon get fixed up alright. Hoping you and baby are well and happy. I will say bye, bye.

Still in Belgium, Harry writes with definite news of his upcoming schedule. He will be back in England and entitled to five days' leave by the middle of February. They hope to sail for Canada by the middle of March. If Iva gets this letter in time, he asks her to cable him some money so he can enjoy his last leave. Things are moving along well and he will soon be home.

January 18, 1919
Estaimbourg, Belgium,

My Dear Wife,

I never had a letter from you for quite a long while but I know you write dear. Just the same we got definite orders yesterday as to when we are going home. We will be in England about the 15th of February and we are going to get five days leave before we sail for Canada. Hon, when you get this letter, if it is not too late, will you cable me some money to go on pass with? We will be sailing for Canada along the first part of March and if you get this letter around the 15th of February or the 20th it will not be too late to cable some money. We are going back to old Bramshott Camp again. Well sweetheart, my fingers are pretty cold writing this letter so you will have to excuse me if I don't write much. I was just talking to Allan a few minutes ago. He is fine. I am well and hope you and baby are the same.

I guess I will close dear for now, so bye, bye, hoping to see you soon, your young husband

Harry's next letter comes a month later. He is back in England and also back from leave, which happened earlier than expected. All is fine, however, for leave cost him very little. Travel in England was free for the troops, and he was treated well by the Newshams at Manchester. Iva did send money, which he received upon his return. His words about the difficulty of keeping any souvenirs for his return are a telling comment on some of his fellow Canadians.

February 18, 1919
Bramshott Camp

My Dear Wife,

I just got back from leave and I had a good time. I was down to Manchester to Mr Newsham's for a whole week. They used me fine. I got the money order today. We went on leave sooner than I thought so the money was too late coming but it didn't cost me anything at Manchester. I had a letter from you today but it was an old one wrote before Christmas. All the same I was glad to get it. I hope to be back home before long. As far as we know, we will be going to Canada somewhere along the first of March. I will try and bring, my dear, some souvenirs home but it is so hard to keep anything around here. We have to keep anything like that in our pockets all the time or it will be stolen. So you see I haven't much chance to get much. Well dear, I hope you and baby are well and happy and all the rest also. I got little Earl's letter today and will answer it as soon as I can. I am feeling fine these days and every day seems like a week because we are waiting to go home. Well dear, I guess I will close as news is very scarce around here, but I will have so much to tell you when I get back.

Harry pens his last letter home to Iva in late February. The army had issued him some new clothes, but in the usual manner: one of each for each man, irrespective of size. His coat would fit their baby, while the hat is very large. He is still concerned about the flu, but focuses on the positive. He will let her know as soon as he reaches the Island. He also mentions the separation pay he will receive, and how much he is looking forward to their reunion and to time spent alone together.

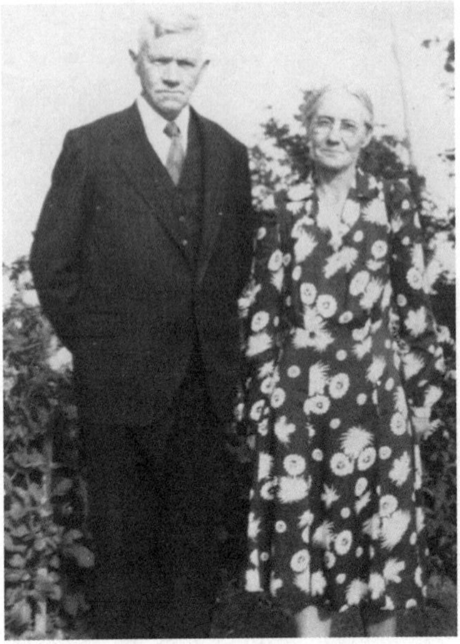

Harry and Iva Mae in old age.

February 23, 1919
Bramshott Camp

My Dear Wife,

Just a line dear to let you know that I am still here but about to be heading for Canada in about a week's time. Believe me I won't be sorry. I saw Allan today, he just came from London last night. His papers are not fixed up yet and I don't know if he will get away with the Battalion or not. I got a new coat and cap last night and I had a good laugh at them. I wish you could see them. The coat is about big enough for our baby and the cap is big enough for Peter Quigly. I am going to try and get them changed tomorrow. There is quite a lot of flu here but I didn't get it yet. I got a few souvenirs for you and baby but I hardly knew what to get. Hope you are all well and happy. Will we be able to go to our little house as soon as I get home? I would rather go home right off as soon as I landed. You will get a telegram as soon as I land, at the expense of the Government. I guess I will have to go to Charlottetown before I get home to turn in my rifle and equipment. I will call you once I reach Charlottetown so you will know. Dear if you will be as glad to see your old man as I will be to see my sweetheart. We will sure be happy. I will be expecting good checks coming too. I will get $100 a month for three months and $35 extra for a suit of clothes. That isn't too bad is it dear? I hope you will be able to come out home whenever I arrive dear as I have so much to tell you. We want to be alone dear. I guess I will close, hoping you are both well and hoping to see you soon.

I will say bye, bye sweetheart, Harry. Guess this will be the last letter if all goes well. I got the baby a gold broach.

Harry's file reveals that he landed in Halifax on March 9, and was formally discharged from the army on March 15, 1919. Harry then went home to Iva and the little fisherman. Harry returned to fishing. He and Iva would have six more children: Lloyd, Earl, Harry Jr, Irene, Francis, and Jean. Harry's son Earl would serve in his generation in the infantry in the Second World War. He saw action in both Italy and northwest Europe and was for a short time a prisoner of war. Sadly, he returned home only to suffer ill health, and died early on March 1, 1947. Harry and Iva continued to live in Summerside. Harry died on February 15, 1967, in his seventy-ninth year. Iva lived until 1981.

Selected Bibliography

Clint, Mabel B. *Our Bit: Memories of War Service by a Canadian Nursing Sister.* Montreal: Barwick, 1934.

Dewar, Katherine. *Called to Serve: Georgina Pope—Canadian Military Nursing Heroine.* Charlottetown: Island Studies Press, 2018.

———. *Those Splendid Girls: The Heroic Service of Prince Edward Island Nurses in the Great War: 1914–1918.* Charlottetown: Island Studies Press, 2014.

Glassford, Sarah, and Amy Shaw. *A Sisterhood of Suffering and Service: Women and Girls of Canada and Newfoundland during the First World War.* Vancouver: UBC Press, 2012.

Mann, Susan. *Margaret Macdonald: Imperial Daughter.* Montreal; Kingston, ON: McGill-Queen's University Press, 2005.

———. *The War Diary of Clare Gass: 1915–1919.* Montreal; Kingston, ON: McGill-Queen's University Press, 2000.

McKenzie, Andrea. *War-Torn Exchanges: The Lives and Letters of Nursing Sisters Laura Holland and Mildred Forbes.* UBC Press: Vancouver, 2014.

Nicholson, G.W.L. *Canada's Nursing Sisters.* Toronto: A.M. Hakkert, 1975.

Quinn, Shawna. *Agnes Warner and the Nursing Sisters of the Great War.* Fredericton, NB: Goose Lane Editions, 2010.

Theobald, Andrew. *The Bitter Harvest of War: New Brunswick and the Conscription Crisis of 1917.* Fredericton, NB: Goose Lane Editions, 2008.

Toman, Cynthia. *Sister Soldiers of the Great War: The Nurses of the Canadian Army Medical Corps.* Vancouver: UBC Press, 2016.

Wilson-Simmie, Katharine. *Lights Out: The Memoir of Nursing Sister Kate Wilson, Canadian Army Medical Corps.* Ottawa: CEF Books, 2004.